What Chiropractic can do for you

Robert Jan Blom

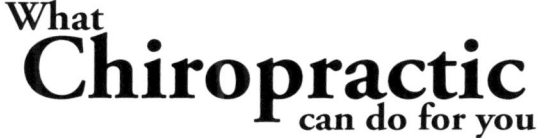

What Chiropractic can do for you

*Natural and safe treatment
of back, shoulders, headache,
migraine and many other symptoms*

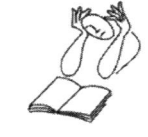

Uitgeverij Aspekt

What Chiropractic can do for you
© Robert Jan Blom
© 2015 Uitgeverij ASPEKT
Amersfoortsestraat 27, 3769 AD Soesterberg, The Netherlands
info@uitgeverijaspekt.nl – http://www.uitgeverijaspekt.nl

Cover Thomas Wunderink
Inside: Uitgeverij Aspekt
Translation: Prof. Dr. James G. Defares

ISBN: 9789461538215
NUR: 180

All rights reserved. No reproduction copy or transmission of this publication may be made without written permission.

Contents

	Introduction	11
1.	**What is chiropractic?**	**21**
	The functioning of the nervous system is disrupted	23
	About health and disturbance	25
2.	**History of Chiropractic**	**28**
	The founder	29
	Opposition of conventional medicine to chiropractic	32
3.	**The human body and chiropractic principles**	**35**
	Not an opponent of conventional medicine	35
	Somewhere something has gone out of balance	38
	The nervous system and the locomotor apparatus	39
4.	**The nervous system**	**40**
	That part we call the sub-consciousness	41
	The central nervous system	43
	The brain	43
	The spinal cord	45
	The peripheral nervous system	45
	The autonomic nervous system	45
	The nerves	47
5.	**The locomotor apparatus**	**48**
	Main characteristic of the locomotor apparatus	49
	For example: the knee meniscus	51
6.	**Disturbance of the nervous system**	**53**
	The condition of the body determines the reaction	55
	Causes of subluxation	56
	Mechanical causes	56
	Psychic causes	59
	Chemical causes	61
	Other causes	62
7.	**To the chiropractor**	**63**
	In the waiting room	64
	Case history and discussion	65

	The physical examination	67
	Whether displaced vertebrae are visible or palpable….	68
	Much depends on the condition of the patient	71
8.	**The treatment**	**72**
	The pressure can be light, sometimes heavier	72
	No pain	73
	The response to adjustments	74
	The human body is difficult to fathom	75
	The Chiropractor is not a miracle doctor	76
	After the treatment	77
9.	**Sport and chiropractic**	**79**
	Common injuries	80
	Neck injuries	80
	Shoulder injuries	80
	Arm injuries	81
	Elbow injuries	81
	Wrists	81
	Hands and feet	81
	Back injuries	81
	Tail bone	81
	Abdominal muscles	82
	Knee	82
	Ankles	82
	Feet and toes	82
	Summary of common sport injuries	82
	How to prevent sport injuries	83
	Training	83
	Minor and serious injuries	84
	The chiropractic treatment	84
10.	**Children and chiropractic**	**85**
	Apparently harmless incidents	86
	When to visit a chiropractor with your child?	88
	The treatment	88
11.	**Pregnancy and chiropractic**	**90**
	Negative effects on the vertebra of the baby	90
12.	**Elderly people and chiropractic**	**92**
	Aching joints	93
	Frozen shoulder	94
	Headache and neck pain	94

	Decalcification of the vertebrae (osteoporosis)	94
	Ankle-knee and wrist ache	94
	Pain below the shoulder blade	95
	Degenerative diseases	95
	Facial neuralgia	96
	And cancer…?	96
	Severe back symptoms	97
	Posture and exercise	97
	Summary common symptoms	98
13.	**Stress and chiropractic**	**99**
	Structural elements in our environment	99
	The nervous system	101
	The environment	101
	The symptoms	102
	Symptoms of stress	102
	A chiropractic idea	103
	What can the chiropractor do?	105
14.	**Most common pains and chiropractic**	**107**
	Backache is not a disease	107
	Sciatica	109
	Other symptoms	110
	Neck, shoulder and arm pains	111
	Headache	112
	The deeper cause	113
	Migraine	114
	What is migraine?	114
	Most common symptoms	115
15.	**The training of the chiropractor**	**116**
	Theoretical subjects combined with practical subjects	117
	Next to the subjects chosen	117
	Study package	118
	Summary prerequisite classes	122
16.	**Movements within chiropractic**	**123**
	Straight or mixed?	123
	Modern variant	124
	Specialisations	125
17.	**Summary: which symptoms?**	**127**
	Low-back symptoms	128
	Anatomy of the back	128

	Upper back and shoulder symptoms	129
	Neck and shoulder complaints	131
	Migraine	133
	Headache	135
	Arthritis – wear	136
	Hernia	138
	Whiplash	142
	Baby's	144
	Children	147
	Pregnancy	148
	Sport injuries	150
18.	**Vertebrae, intervertebral disks and possible complaints**	**152**
19.	**What chiropractic is not**	**159**
	Osteopathy	159
	The osteopath tries to restore the original structure	162
	Manual medicine	163
	Manual therapy: 'system-Sickesz'	165
	Manual therapy: 'system Van der Bijl'	167
20.	**Preventing symptoms yourself**	**169**
	Preventing backache	169
	Neck-, shoulder- and arm pain	171
	Headache complaints and migraine	172
21.	**Diet and health**	**174**
	What exactly is poor and what is healthy food?	175
	Meat or no meat, that's the question…	175
	Bircher Benner- diet	177
	Mayr-cure	178
	The diet	180
	Macrobiotics	181
	Eating and drinking differently	182
	Sugar	182
	Salt	183
	Coffee	183
	And other drugs?	183
22.	**Breathing**	**185**
	Oxygen	185
	Exercise	186
	Complaints	187

23	**With nature together**	**188**
	Concern about one's own life-style	188
	Think positive	190
	Opening the door to nature	191
	Disease must also be seen as a warning	192
24.	**Most frequently asked questions about chiropractic**	**195**
Glossary		**201**

Introduction

From a dark period, dominated by spirits, gods and demons

'Disease was mostly a punishment and only since the 16th century people understood that healing had to be promoted'

The functioning of the human body has been observed for thousands of years. Still the body divulged few of its secrets. It's true much had to be discovered, but no one knew where to begin with that voyage of discovery. What did one know about the human body, about illness and health? Of course the Chinese, the Greek and the Romans did their best and even today it still holds that they made important contributions to medicine. But if one looks at their advances scientifically the results are disappointing.

And after the fall of the Roman Empire (476 A.D.) the progress of medical knowledge virtually came to a halt.

It was not until the year 1030 that the Persian scholar Ibn Sina (980-1037) published his medical standard work the *Canon Medicinae*, an encyclopaedia dealing with infectious diseases and mental conditions like insomnia and melancholia. Ibn Sina also wrote about anatomy, physiology and surgery. In the five volumes of this work two discoveries were described that are still topical today: the high sugar level in the urine of diabetics and the fact that water should be boiled in the treatment of infectious diseases.

Despite this important step on the laborious road of medical science progress came to a halt and a new age dawned in which the quack prevailed and fables and rumours ran rampant, times known, with regard to disease and health, as the centuries of folk medicine. A long and dark period dominated by spirits, gods and demons. Today we sometimes laugh about those times and contemptuously dismiss those old wives' tales. Still we should not ignore those times that were after all also important in the development of medical knowledge.

Every fairy tale, as well as every new 'medicine' in those days was a step on the road to what is now called conventional medicine. Despite all the strange medical excesses of those times folk medicine constituted the conventional medicine of its day.

Anger of the gods or dominance of demons
Information about the slowly progressing art of healing and the knowledge about the human body came sparingly and was confined to certain regions or districts. There were no publications in those days, no scientific studies and so, no transmission of knowledge existed. Seekers of the secrets of the human body understood this and continued to puzzle about the causes of illness, studied the human body and developed theories to save the life of the diseased person and to extend it. Alas, few answers to medical questions turned out to exist, as a result of which intangible solutions such as a higher power, like gods or demons, were often invoked. So-called *wise men* were called upon to mediate between the sick and the higher power. Heal-

ing was 'invoked' and when that failed to occur that pointed to anger of the gods or the predominance of demons. The Germans appointed '*wise women*' (Saga's) who served to exorcise demons and appease the gods. With insanity it was important to drive away the evil spirits and when one fainted the soul must have fled, so it was argued. Disease was a matter of fate, mostly a punishment and only since the 16th century people realized that diseases could also be influenced by humans and, so, healing could be promoted.

Despite this, in those days 'new way of thinking', little changed and quacks continued to occupy an important place in folk medicine. 'Horoscoper' and 'pill peddlers' dominated medicine. Until the 19th century it was believed that you could make someone ill by for example drawing a nail through the eye on a statuette representing the other person. Or it was thought that disease could be transferred to others or to animals, resulting in a cure. Rheumatism was treated by letting a dog sleep near the affected joints. Sick children or children crying a lot were 'cured' by giving them a different name. Sore throat disappeared after the 'healer' held a frog in front of the open mouth. The frog would then take over the sore throat. Disease demons lived in animals and diseases with fever were ascribed to demons living in the dog (in Dutch German measles is still called '*red dog*'). Warts disappeared after being touched by the hand of a corpse…..And warts could also be 'sold', a belief that persisted till far into the 20th century. The exorcism of evil spirits still goes on to this day, while many other forms of treatment also stem directly from views held in those times.

> *'Disease demons lived in animals and
> disorders with fever were ascribed
> to demons living in the dog'*

It was not until the 19th century, that a change occurred. Only those who had studied at a medical university were allowed to practise medicine. From that year on medicine was moving in a different direction with, however, little promise of change. For the common man it turned out that even after World War 2 it was virtually impossible to benefit from the latest developments in medicine.

The common cold still cannot be prevented
It is true that science developed at a fair pace. For many symptoms solutions were found in the 20th century. But it is clear that we still have a long way to go. A simple common cold can still not be prevented. Although many forms of cancer can be cured today, the disease is still as much feared as the plague in the middle-ages.

Moreover, man will always be threatened by new diseases. Aids is a case in point. Today cardio-vascular diseases are reasonably under control, but these conditions still constitute the most important causes of death. But the search goes on for new solutions, new methods and new medicines.

> *'He is received and handled by people
> in white coats, people without a face'*

As was noted at the beginning of this introduction, man and his health had been the focus of attention for centuries. Despite the progress in medicine the individual is in danger of fading into the background. Now the main thing is the disease. The individual behind the illness is largely ignored. Medicine is being flooded by a plethora of available drugs. The patient is fully aware of it and feels abandoned by his family doctor or specialist. He/she feels isolated in a room full of medical instruments, as he is being received and handled by 'people in white coats, people without a face'.

The treatment method often feels cold and impersonal. Remember that a sick person is also a person in distress. With palpable fear of the consequences of the disease, sometimes fear of death, something one hardly dares to think about but thrusts itself upon the mind.

A sick person needs attention, understanding and warm heartedness, matters you usually won't get from your family doctor or specialist. There are after all still so many patients in the waiting rom. The doctor has little time, is forced to work quickly. He has been taught to treat disorders; he has not been taught to pay attention to the person behind the disease, the person who sorely needs his attention and empathy. The doctor has also been taught that symptoms establish the presence of the disease and when the symptoms disappear the disease will be cured. In a negative sense it is called *treatment of symptoms*. Although I definitely have no negative attitude towards conventional medicine and sympathise with the well-meaning doctor I regret the fact that within the scope of the fast expanding medical developments the disease is the main focus of attention.

The human body is a complicated 'engine'
As mentioned the patient feels more or less abandoned and is aware that this treatment of symptoms not always offer the solution. A telling comparison is when an engine gets jammed it doesn't happen without a reason. It must have an underlying cause. Perhaps a part of the engine is worn out, of too little attention had been given to the engine. So, the motor is in need of repairs, but a repair can never be properly carried out as long as the cause of the defect has not been identified.

The human body must be viewed in the same way. When something goes wrong, when a disease is present, it means that something has gone wrong, that too little attention has been paid to the body. Recovery is only possible when the cause is found, just as with the engine. An engine doesn't get jammed 'just like that', an illness doesn't occur 'just like that'. Every dysfunction has a cause. An engine is not really complicated, but the human body is the most complicated 'engine' you can imagine.

Eastern cultures have realized for thousands of years that a cause lies hidden behind every disease. Eastern healers thus concentrate on that cause and only thereafter on the actual disorder. In our society it is often the other way round. The disease is present; the symptoms show it. The disease is treated with drugs which have been shown to be effective and from which a positive result can be expected. But long ago man has discovered that nature offers us drugs from plants. People are part of nature and with what nature has to offer diseases often can be cured. In our technological society we are often in too much hurry to produce drugs from plants. We also can't wait for a good harvest of plants that can contribute to our health.

So, we have experimented until we were able to produce synthetic drugs with the same action as the plants of former days. The body is being pounded with chemicals, or rather, the disorder is being 'bombarded' by these substances.

The disease fights a battle with chemicals and it is hoped that the disease loses this battle. But, since the cause of the disorder is not addressed, there is always a risk that the symptoms will return with the passage of time. Then, more chemicals are required. Maybe they win the battle with the disorder but the body cannot handle all those chemicals. We consume food with colourings and flavourings, sprayed vegetables and fruit, while factories belch chemical substances that we inhale every day. On top of that there are the exhaust fumes from cars, perhaps we smoke, work too hard, take too little exercise and are under great stress. We are on a treadmill without end. Or, are we…?

*'The body is being pounded by chemicals,
or rather, the disorder is being 'bombarded' by these substances'*

Many no longer accept what the doctor prescribes. Patients are looking for a safer method so that the already sick body is not further exposed to harmful chemicals. We ask critical questions and are no longer convinced that his view is the only valid one. A bright spot is that the healthy individual is looking for ways to stay in good health, even by drastically changing his or her lifestyle. People again try to connect with nature. We have almost forgotten that we are part of nature and are asking nature to lead us the way. In there is no room for chemicals, tranquilizers or sleeping pills and rather no drugs in general.

We are on the right track and slowly society appears to be changing. Not all doctors reject other than conventional forms of treatment. An increasing number realizes that a cause and a human being are behind the disorder. There are visible signs of this hesitant change. Insurance companies are willing to reimburse the costs of alternative treatments and some doctors even refer the patient to alternative therapists.

There is more than just the treatment of symptoms…
Our view on sickness and health was bound to change if one realizes that about twenty percent of the adult population visits an alternative therapist or uses an alternative medicine, e.g. homeopathic home remedies. Patients are aware that conventional medicine won't bring universal happiness either and that there is more than just the treatment of symptoms, despite the spectacular progress of conventional medicine.

He/she who opens his/her mind to other views and seeks expert advice or treatment by an alternative therapist is faced with a problem. To whom should I turn ? Who can help me? Which treatment is best suited for my condition? Which therapist is the right therapist? There are so many methods, so many therapists and so many treatments. We can't see the wood for the trees.

Chiropractic, by now a well-known and popular therapy
This book deals with chiropractic and sheds light on a by-now well-known and popular therapy. Chiropractic comprises diagnosis, treatment and prevention of certain disorders. Most symptoms treated by the chiropractor involve the back, the shoulders and the neck. Headache, migraine, facial pain and tingling or numbness in arms or legs may be present. Pain and stiffness, e.g. from arthritis (wear) may be greatly reduced by chiropractic. Women with low back pain during pregnancy or with menstrual pain may benefit from chiropractic.

Symptoms originating outside the spine can be treated as well: sore muscles, painful joints, e.g. the elbows, knees, ankles and feet. Even with arthritis pain relief and functional improvement can sometimes be achieved. As the organs and tissues of the body require an undisturbed nerve supply it should be evident that many functional disorders are favourably affected by chiropractic. This applies as well to vague symptoms like dizziness, tiredness and listlessness: sometimes the cause is found to be in the spinal column.

A chiropractor is a 'professional' certified in many European countries, including many member states of the European Union, to practise his profession. In the USA and Canada chiropractic is currently one of the three most popular forms of treatment. In these countries chiropractic occupies third place, after conventional medicine and dentistry. Chiropractors have received their training in colleges in the USA, Brazil, South-Africa, Australia, Canada, England, France, Spain, Denmark or Switzerland.

About this book
All posible aspects of chiropractic are discussed in this book: what exactly chiropractor entails, what the chiropractor can do for his/her patients, about the training of the chiropractor. A practical and useful book for anyone aiming for optimal health or desires to be cured from an disorder without medicines or operation.

This book describes how the healthy person can prevent symptoms and how the sick person can be treated by the chiropractor. He who makes use of the chiropractic view on disease and health can experience personally that health and disease can be viewed from a different perspective. From the chiropractic viewpoint for example ….

Robert Jan Blom
Author

1. What is chiropractic?

'By way of the nerves the impulses arrive at the organs and tissues. There the body functions are regulated'

Chiropractic is a holistic form of healing that attempts to promote, to restore and to support the total health of the individual by restoring the breakdown in communication in the functioning of the nervous system through the application of a measured mechanical impulse. The chiropractor does not use surgery and/or radiation.

Body functions, organs and tissues operate through vital nerve impulses from the brain that run via the spinal-cord and the nerve endings. Via a complicated neural network nerve energy-impulses literally sustain life. It is well-established that the nervous system controls the whole body. The nervous system is comprised of the central nervous system, brain, spinal cord and nerves. These subdivisions of the nervous system are, of course, intimately linked.

The brain produces the required energy and this is transmitted as electrical impulses via the spinal cord that emerge at certain points between the vertebrae. Via the nerves these impulses arrive at the organs and tissues. There the body functions are regulated.

The brain continuously receives information from the organs and tissues, information about their functioning and the environment in which the organs operate. This information is processed and produces an almost instantaneous response. The nervous system provides 'action and reaction'. In this the spinal-column plays a crucial role. As was noted before the nerve impulses are transmitted via the spinal cord enclosed and protected by the spinal column. The spinal column consists of a number of bones -vertebrae- that serve to protect this very delicate transmission process but these bones may also obstruct the passage of nerve energy to the organs.

Picture 1

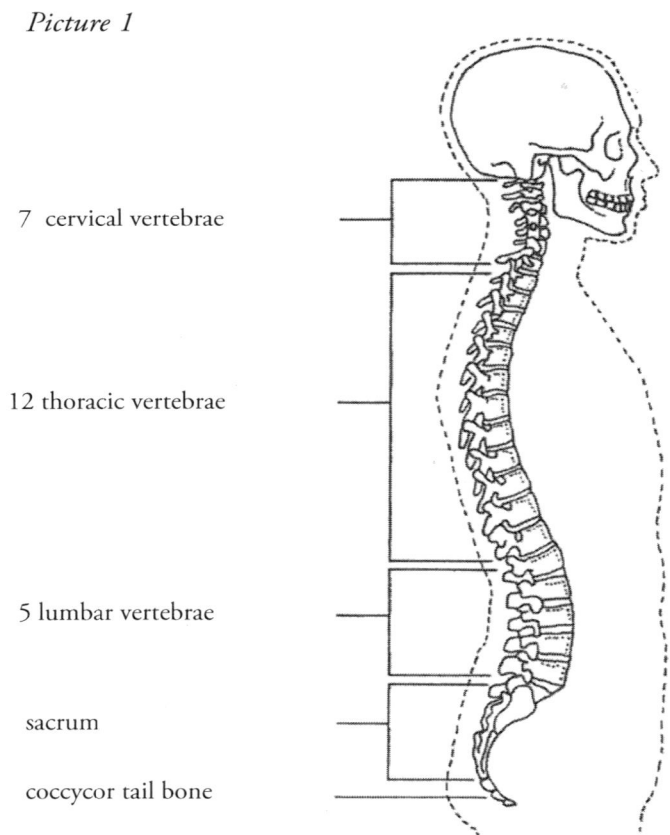

7 cervical vertebrae

12 thoracic vertebrae

5 lumbar vertebrae

sacrum

coccycor tail bone

The functioning of the nervous system is disrupted
The spinal column consists of 7 cervical vertebrae, 12 thoracic vertebrae, 5 lumbar vertebrae, the sacrum and the coccyx or tailbone (see picture 1). This bony structure is moving all the time. By various causes it may happen that the movement between two vertebrae is impeded. Then the proper functioning of the nervous system is disrupted. This can cause local pain, but the blocked vertebrae may also pinch nerves as a result of which the supply of nerve energy to the organs and tissues is disrupted. The blocked nerves are also irritated which usually causes pain. But now the organs and tissues no longer receive sufficient energy. It is thus obvious that these organs no longer function optimally. It may be that the organ functions sub-optimally or virtually not at all. In other words: it is a matter of a disorder or symptoms. From this it follows that recovery is only possible when the blockade can be removed, thereby removing the resulting disturbance in the nervous system and thus restoring the energy supply.

When this is achieved, then the organs that had thus far been deprived of energy, regain the energy they need to function normally. Usually recovery occurs after correction of the blockade. The pinching of nerves by a mobility disturbance is called *subluxation*.

This term will be used in this book a number of times.

This theory thus posits that disorders and symptoms do not occur as long as the vertebrae in the spinal-column are not blocked and thus do not press on the nerves (or pinch them), thus allowing the nervous system to perform optimally. The theory implies that diseases result from pinching or irritation of nerve fibres .

The question whether diseases can also derive from other causes will be discussed in chapter 16, entitled, "Movements within chiropractic'.
In any case the theory maintains that as a result of subluxation disorders can be caused (as well as pain), a theory which is the foundation of chiropractic. On the basis of the above it also follows that the chiropractor is not directly engaged in curing diseases. The chiropractor concentrates on correcting a disturbance within the nervous system enabling the body itself to cure the disorder. In the view of the chiropractor the body possesses the innate wisdom to keep the body free of diseases, to ward off 'attacks from outside'. The term 'innate wisdom' can also be translated as 'life force', or 'body consciousness'.

> *'The body possesses a certain 'intelligence' enabling it to respond to stimuli'*

This innate wisdom or 'innate intelligence' is closely linked to the 'vital life force', which in its turn is connected to man's spiritual force. According to ancient tradition it was believed that these reached the body through the 'life veins' from which the nervous system derives its force. Others, too, within the medical community share this view. In short, the body possesses a certain 'intelligence' enabling it to respond to stimuli. When it concerns attacks that can make the body sick it responds adequately. The intelligence regulates all vital functions, indirectly also the intellectual part within us. The chiropractor greatly respects the innate wisdom of the body. So there is no need to interfere by the administration of drugs or surgery. Nota bene: this concerns the basic principles of chiropractic. When the chiropractor has no solution to offer then he will certainly refer the patient to another therapist, family doctor or specialist.

> **Mixed chiropractic**
> The 'mixed' chiropractors constitute the modern variety. They mix other techniques in their therapy, make as far as possible a diagnosis and do not limit themselves to correcting subluxations. Indeed, the terms 'subluxation' and 'innate intelligence' (life force) derived from the Palmer's original theories are considered to be unscientific and incomplete. Mixed chiropractors are open to a professional dialogue and have the ambition to attain a recognized position within conventional medicine. Mixed chiropractors are more nuanced in their claims about effectiveness and restrict their sphere of activity to symptoms of the locomotor apparatus, such as low back pain, neck pain, headaches, sport injuries, etc. No claims are made about its effectiveness concerning organic disorders and other pathological processes.
> **See chapter 16;** *Trends within chiropractic*

About health and disturbance

Despite that innate wisdom of the body itself, a *mechanical defect* may occur: the subluxation.

The result is a blocked vertebra that pinches the nerve, by which the nervous system can no longer operate optimally, resulting in damage to the organs. When the nervous system does not work optimally organs and tissues are unable to function optimally. This gives cause for the chiropractor to act. At the beginning of this chapter we had already said that the treatment is aimed at restoring breakdown in communication within the nervous system. This is done by the hands and sometimes instruments are used. The spinal-column constitutes an important link with regard to our health. Thus, the chiropractor mainly concentrates on the spinal-column.

After chiropractic correction the energy again flows through the complex nervous system and again reaches the organs and tissues to a sufficient degree. The nervous energy is once more brought into proper balance. Disorders and symptoms disappear as does, of course, the pain. The pain manifests itself in the first place at the site of the displaced vertebra, but may also occur at other locations. The patient may, besides backache, also complain of neck and shoulder pain, while headache or general malaise may be present.

The definition of chiropractic correction involves that the chiropractor aims at adjusting dislocated vertebrae and adhesions, by which nerve disturbances are corrected. *The innate intelligence,* or innate wisdom acting in the human body can once again fulfil its duty to bring about a new balance in the body and restore the normal state of harmony and health. The state of health then simply excludes pain and disease.

Summary of the basic principles:
- The body possesses the ability to protect itself against diseases. With this the correct functioning of the nervous system is of vital importance.

- In consequence of a mechanical disturbance (subluxation) within the spinal-column the passage of nerve impulses from and towards the brain can be negatively affected. The nervous system then does not function optimally.
- The disturbance of the nervous system and the diminished action of the nerves constitute the most important cause of disease and symptoms (including pain).
- It is the job of the chiropractor to remove this disturbance within the nervous system by correcting blocked spinal cord segments (vertebrae and discs) by which the disturbance within the nervous system is removed.
- The correction is carried out by hand, without drugs, without radiation, without operation.

2. History of Chiropractic

*'It is necessary to have a thorough knowledge of
the spinal-column, for many disorders are actually
caused by a defect in the spinal-column'*

This quote looks like having been taken from a modern medical textbook. Yet this is not the case. The quotation is from the Greek physician Hippocrates (460-377 BC).

Already that long ago he was convinced that the vertebrae played an important part in the causation of symptoms and poor health. But not only Hippocrates felt that the condition of the spinal–column had to be causally involved to disease. In old Chinese texts of some five thousand years ago manipulations are described reminiscent of modern chiropractic. And in ancient Greek papyrus texts dating from 1500 BC the connection between disease and the condition of the spinal-column is mentioned. In South -and Central America were Indian tribes who in disease let themselves be beaten on the back by sacks filled with wet seeds. Also children were made to walk on the back of the sick person as 'treatment' for various ailments.

Throughout the centuries the idea was developed that the vertebrae played a decisive role in health and disease and that symptoms were causally related to the state of the spinal-column. Much of the accumulated knowledge that might be considered 'scientific' was lost with the fall of the Roman Empire (476 AD).

From that time on superstition and the belief in evil spirits and demons held sway for centuries (the dark middle-ages). Despite this, people continued to push this idea and remained convinced that the spinal-column held the key to health and disease. Physicians, too, turned their mind in those ancient times on the spinal-column and performed medical manipulations sometimes resulting in a cracking sound. This was interpreted as exorcism. Today chiropractors are sometimes irreverently called *bone crackers*.

The founder
In 1845 Daniel David Palmer was born. Despite his great interest in the human body and 'things medical' the young Daniel couldn't bring himself to study medicine. First he found a job in fish shops and groceries. Later Daniel held a job as teacher in business knowledge. Outside his job he keeps himself occupied with the studying the functioning of the human body. He studies phrenology, a discarded form of character analysis based on the study of the skull. He gives lectures on the subject. At one of these talks he meets the magnetizer Paul Caster. He has a great admiration for Caster, who, in his turn is sympathetic towards the young Palmer. Carter passes on his knowledge to Palmer and after a couple of years Palmer starts his own magnetizer practice in Burlington (USA). Besides his work he studies anatomy and physiology. He then becomes convinced that the spinal-column is of far greater importance than had thus far been suspected. Palmer proposes that the human body is provided with nervous energy via the spinal-column and that

that nervous supply is blocked by pinching from displacements of vertebrae. He strongly suspects that this pinching could very well be the cause of symptoms hitherto unconnected to the condition of spinal-column.

At a certain moment Palmer came to the conclusion that he possessed sufficient knowledge of the human body to call himself *doctor,* at the time an unprotected title. As a *physician* he further developed his theories, invented the name *chiropractic* and puts his philosophy and method of treatment in writing. By that time Daniel David Palme is fifty years old and chiropractic is only practised by him. That did not satisfy Palmer and in 1897 he starts offering three months courses. The *'Palmer Infirmary and Chiropractic School'* is established in Davenport, Iowa (USA) and the course turns out to be a great success. Among the many students are doctors, surgeons and osteopaths, among whom Dr. Alfred E. Walton of the University of Pennsylvania. He would later bring chiropractic to the attention of the established medical community in the United States.

> *'Throughout the centuries people developed the idea that symptoms were related to the condition of the spinal-column'*

Among Palmer's students were two young individuals who would later raise chiropractic to unprecedented popularity. First, his son Bartlett Joshua Palmer (1881) and Mabel Heath. Both students fall in love with each other and decide to marry. But for father, son and Mabel many setbacks still lie ahead. Although the foundation had been laid and the interest is growing opposition against chiropractic from conventional medicine is spreading. Palmer and his son are accused of improperly practicing medicine. In 1906 both men are arrested, a setback and serious humiliation.

Undeterred, the Palmers continue on their chosen path. The number of training schools are expanded and in the states of Oklahoma and Oregon colleges for chiropractic education are founded. In 1913 Daniel David Parker dies. Bartlett takes over his father's job while his wife Mabel gives instruction in one of the schools founded by Daniel.

Despite his sensational view on sickness and health, training courses and his Chiropractic Schools Daniel David Palmer died as a relatively unknown person. But shortly after his death his *invention* is recognized in Kansas and North-Dakota and seven years later, in 1920, chiropractic is recognized in 24 of the 48 American states! At the time dozens of universities already offer courses in chiropractic and a number of foundations have been founded: The International Chiropractic Association and The American Chiropractic Association among others. But in those days the students too developed their own vision of the ideas proposed by Bartlett Palmer. Whereas Bartlett's notions strictly conformed to his father's, students believed that causes other than subluxation could cause disease. Even to this day differences of opinion (albeit small) within the chiropractic community exist (see chapter 16 *Trends within Chiropractic*). For example, the founder and his son were unwilling to use instruments for determining abnormalities inside the spinal-column. Even the use of the *spinograph*, an X-ray instrument introduced in 1909, encountered resistance from the followers of Daniel and Bartlett Palmer.

Opposition of conventional medicine to chiropractic
It is true that a few years later Bartlett accepted the *spinograph* but this created a rift with those of his students who strictly subscribed to the ideas of the older Palmer. So chiropractic struggled on until 1933.In that year a new instrument was introduced, the *neurocalometer,* a true sensation in its day. The instrument enabled the chiropractor to measure temperature differences at both sides of the spinal-column, something that greatly facilitated locating disturbances in the nervous system. Even the conservative Bartlett allowed the use of the instrument, thereby arousing the ire of the group that strictly adhered to the basic principles laid down by Daniel Palmer.

In the meantime the war of conventional medicine against chiropractic continued unabated. The scientists were strongly opposed to chiropractors being allowed to take medical finals, despite the fact that most American states recognized chiropractic which was taught at many colleges. Because of this the scientists' protests were ineffective and in 1930 chiropractic students were permitted to take medical finals. But many of these students chose to strike out on a different medical course after graduating, to the detriment of chiropractic. This became such a problem that many chiropractic colleges were closed down. Mabel Palmer-Smith died in 1949, while her husband, Bartlett Palmer passed away in 1961.

Despite the many setbacks it was impossible to imagine life in America without chiropractic and its popularity continued to grow. The quality of instruction improved while the scientific study about the effectiveness of chiropractic finally got off the ground. In the seventies the Health Department (USA) recognized chiropractic and a grant of $ 2 million dollars was made available for scientific studies. Congress added the 'new treatment' to the *medical program*, while in 1975 the outcome of the scientific study resulted in chiropractors being placed at the same level as regular doctors.

In the USA chiropractic occupies third place after regular medicine and dentistry. Today chiropractic is also officially recognized in Canada, New-Zeeland, Bolivia, Switzerland and, of course, in the USA. In Australia, England, Venezuela, Peru and scores of other countries chiropractors have been allowed to practise for years.

'In the USA chiropractic occupies third place after regular medicine and dentistry'

In Holland and Belgium hundreds of chiropractors are working and a number of organisations exercise supervision over it. In these countries the authorities have thus far not formally recognized chiropractic.

Chiropractic is, as mentioned above, a fact of life in our society and its value is widely recognized. A treatment which has been in existence for 'merely' 120 years might be referred to as the *new* form of treatment. On the basis of the philosophy and treatment of chiropractic we are actually dealing with a method of treatment whose value has been recognized thousands of years ago.

3. The human body and chiropractic principles

> *'The chiropractor has a different view than the regular physician. This does not mean that all other methods of treatment are rejected by chiropractic'*

In this chapter the question will be answered how chiropractic may contribute to our health. It is of interest to know how our body works and how the chiropractor uses this knowledge. It is fascinating to take a closer look behind the scenes of our own functioning required to understand how chiropractic interprets that functioning in connection with chiropractic principles. The human body is an extremely complex 'machine' with a perfect computer, our brain.

Not an opponent of conventional medicine

Before we discuss the workings of the nervous system the following observation is in order. The current medical technology is highly advanced. With the aid of instruments we can take a close look inside the human body. When we find that an organ has been stricken with a disease the pharmaceutical industry is ready to offer the appropriate drug. Or, doctors reach for instruments to speed up the recovery process. To prevent misunderstandings: the chiropractor is absolutely no opponent of conventional medicine. The developments within medicine have also provided the chiropractor with a better knowledge of the human body. But the chiropractor is flatly opposed to the excessive use of drugs or a too hasty decision to operate. The chiropractor has a very different view than the regular physician. That does not imply that all other methods of treatment are rejected by chiropractic.

The aim of chiropractic is to help the body function optimally. Helping does not mean the prompt prescription of drugs or rash surgery. This is an aim for which the chiropractor earns our respect. In his turn the chiropractor respects regular medicine and its rapid development. About this much can be said.

Conventional medicine has - generally speaking - little regard for chiropractic. But a ray of hope is that mutual respect is growing. We should not forget that both conventional medicine and chiropractic are working for the same cause: the health of the patient. In some situations the chiropractor may decide that it is in the patient's interest to consult his family doctor or a specialist for examination and treatment. In that case the chiropractor will definitely refer the patient to his doctor. Conversely, doctors increasingly refer the patient to the chiropractor. This co-operation is necessary and is a promising development. Whenever people are working on health issues cooperation should be the first priority. Where one fails to find the missing piece of the most complicated puzzle in existence the other may hold it in his hand.

This puzzle is so complicated that it is nonsense to fear that one day technology will replace man. All technology will be guided and controlled by humans. It will never be otherwise.

> *'Conversely, doctors increasingly refer the patient to the chiropractor'*

The chiropractor goes beyond just treating the affected organ or stimulating a poorly functioning organ. The chiropractor posits the inborn wisdom of the body that knows how to respond to symptoms. And who knows how to deal with attacks from outside. The founder of chiropractic, Daniel David Palmer once said, "Every living creature, every human, every animal, every plant possesses innate intelligence. This innate intelligence manifests itself through the nervous system". By that he referred to the capacity of the body to keep itself free of disease and to correct imperfections. That one could call innate wisdom, but one could just as well refer to it as 'nature'. Nature has created us, we are part of nature. So, nature can help us when a disturbance arises.

But nature doesn't mind being assisted or to be reminded of the task to correct imperfections or fight diseases. Due to our life-style a mechanical disturbance may occur. Nature may be temporarily upset as a result. For we no longer live according to the laws and desires of nature. The chiropractor respects the emphatic desire of nature to correct the defects itself. For the chiropractor who loves to help nature this respect remains great. The innate wisdom of the body is then gently awakened, even disciplined, after which nature continues its course.

This is one of the most important principles of chiropractic. Not to interfere in nature with artificial substances or unnatural methods. Just helping nature a bit, asking it to continue with the important action of this innate intelligence. That's all and nature shows its gratitude for this *simple signal*. That nature listens to this signal is shown by the good results obtained by the chiropractor. Nature responds, resumes its proper job and promotes recovery of the affected organs or restores their harmonious functioning.

Somewhere something has gone out of balance
In this book it is made clear that disease is not an isolated event. Disease means there is something wrong or something has gone wrong with the whole body. The organs in the body are interdependent and the interplay between organs and organ functions makes man such a complicated but perfect whole. Those who look at only one organ and treat, that one organ in fact deny the perfect connection between all organs and functions. But once again, this cannot be held against conventional medicine. Technology will always be controlled by humans but sometimes it may outstrip us. We lose our way, also a very human trait. The chiropractor holds fast to nature, follows nature and helps it. Because nature may have lost its way. Man as part of nature has the duty to point this out to nature and to help. That is the task of the chiropractor.

The nervous system and the locomotor apparatus
He who wishes to serve nature must first understand how it works. And since we are talking about the human body we have to understand how the human body is constructed and functions. Not everything is yet known. But we do know that the nervous system controls and regulates the body. Chiropractic starts from this basic truth. The nervous system is especially protected by bony structures: the skull and the spinal column. This protection by the spinal column can be hampered by causes that will be discussed in later chapters. These protective bones may sometimes interfere with the nervous system, cause irritation and obstruction. The chiropractor frees the body from this irritation or obstruction and the nervous system can once again operate freely.

4. The nervous system

*'The idea that one day we shall be controlled
by robots who can do more than
the human brain is a myth'*

In chapter 1 (*What is chiropractic*) it is mentioned that every physical function operates on nervous impulses from the brain and that the nervous system controls the whole body. In order to understand this some knowledge of the nervous system is required. In this chapter this complicated system on which we utterly depend will be discussed. The view of chiropractic rests on the determining role of this system. First we will discuss the nervous system generally and after that the central nervous system and peripheral nervous system.

The nervous system consists of an extremely sophisticated versatile system on which we are utterly dependent. A system whose activity and structure determines our daily life and hence our functioning. The brain is part of it: the human brain which may be called the most versatile, the most perfect *computer* in existence and which can never be replaced by computers.

Technology will never be able to replace the human brain. That is out of the question! The idea that one day we shall be controlled by robots who can do more than the human brain is a myth. The only thing man is able to do will be to develop technologies to which our knowledge can be transferred. But it will always remain our knowledge, originating in our brains.

That part we call the sub-consciousness
Anyway it is firmly established that the brain can do much more than we have hitherto suspected. Possibly we will one day make better use of our brains than we do now. Memory for example is in fact largely terra incognita when we realize that the retrievable memory constitutes but a quarter of our total memory and that the greatest part of our memory is not retrievable. That part we call the subconscious.

In it an unimaginable amount of knowledge is stored, possibly all knowledge that has ever been transferred to man. But we are unable to simply retrieve this knowledge. That huge amount of knowledge remains in the 'sleeping mode' in our subconscious. The fact remains that the subconscious is present and that one day we shall be able to retrieve this 'sleeping' knowledge.

The human nervous system operates *'automatically'*, which justifies the comparison with a computer. Through countless pathways billions of cells communicate with each other. Those cells regulate various functions. For example they control abstract and concrete functions, constructive and destructive functions, bodily and intellectual functions. All these functions are maintained with very little expenditure of energy and are activated by stimuli.

In our memory a *'pattern'* is stored. The brain receives stimuli from 'outside': a new pattern is created that is compared with the pattern in our memory. Sometimes the stimuli the brain receives are numerous. Instantly these new stimuli are selected and assessed. Then an adequate response follows. This instantaneous assessment in the brain may be compared to a carefully thought-out decision. But a decision is preceded by arguments and considerations. The brain does it in a split second. But still the ultimate decision and the subsequent actions are stored in our memory, including the arguments and considerations underlying the decision. So the brain learns from it and adds the experience to the memory pattern. This means that next time a new experience, new stimuli are processed even faster, resulting in the reaction being than the first time. A good analogy is someone taking riding lessons. The pupil is being *bombarded* with new stimuli, new experiences and our memory needs time to turn these experiences into reactions and so into actions. That means that the pupil has to reflect since the new stimuli are not yet part of the pattern stored in memory. But the brain 'remembers' all decisions and acts taken after reflection. Therefore the stimuli will require increasingly less 'reflection time' for processing. After a while the actions to be executed will proceed faster and faster. Now, the actions to be executed are part of the *memory pattern.* Eventually every proceeds so fast that one thinks one can ride a horse or drive a car 'automatically'.

*'A decision is preceded by arguments and considerations.
The brain does it in a split second'*

Decisions are taken on the basis of abstract reasoning and not exclusively on the basis of personal experiences. The brain receives a huge amount of sensory information. Receptors for vision, hearing, smell and touch transmit information to the brain. This information is in fact a packet of instructions spread over the central nerve cells. An adequate response follows and much information is processed automatically, reflexly. Part of it is influenced by the higher centers in the brain. This enables us to make a choice between various alternatives.

The central nervous system
The brain and spinal cord make up the central nervous system. Nerves divide from the spinal column. This system observes the environment and signals changes in it. The body adapts to this. The spinal cord nerves combine the central nervous system with the autonomic nervous system which will be discussed later in this chapter.

The brain
The cerebral cortex, the largest part of the brain consists of two hemispheres. Each hemisphere contains a cavity where cerebrospinal fluid is constantly produced. Via two other cavities the fluid enters the so-called arachnoid space which covers the brain and the spinal cord. At the back of the brain, in front of the cerebellum, lies the pineal gland, a pea-size endocrine gland. Further the thalamus is a very important part of the midbrain, with many im-

portant centres and 'thalamus nuclei'. The nuclei are interconnected and link-up with the cerebral cortex. During every brain activity these thalamus nuclei play a central role. For instance they are closely involved in the sensation of pain, in perception and emotions, while they also play a role in will power and personality.

The cerebellum is located behind the brainstem (the 'head' of the spinal cord) and covered by the hindmost part of the brain. The cerebellum controls body posture and body movements. (see chapter 5. *The locomotor system*). Muscle tone too is regulated by the cerebellum. The midbrain split in front into two parts, while two pair of 'hills' are involved in vision and hearing. The cranial nerves subdivide from the midbrain and exit at various locations. Between the nuclei and nervous fibres of the brainstem which, located above the spinal column turns into the midbrain, is a network of white and grey matter. Many connections exist with other parts of the brain and this matter is probably responsible for heartbeat, respiration and locomotion.

> **The brain**
> The brain consists of a number of parts. Through the spinal cord we enter the skull and encounter the rhombencephalon, consisting of the cerebellum, pons (jutting part of the base of the brain) medulla oblongata ('head' of the spinal cord), the mid-brain (mesencephalon) and the pro-encephalon (in front). The pro-encephalon consists of the telencephalon, the thalamus and the hypothalamus (important centre of nuclei in the diencephalon).

The spinal cord
The spinal cord is that part of the central nervous system protected by the spinal column. It consists of a column of grey matter surrounded by white matter. This matter transmits information to the thalamus, while it also transmits motor signals from the brain to below.

The peripheral nervous system
The word *peripheral* means 'on the outside', so, the peripheral nervous system means the nervous system at the 'outside' of the body (*outside* the central nervous system). The peripheral nervous system connects the central nervous system with the rest of the body. It consists of motor nerves and sensory nerves. Motor nerves are nerves that transmit the impulse to move to the muscles and sensory nerves are sense nerves, e.g. nerves that transmit tactile sensations to the brain. Some of these nerves control the exocrine glands (these, unlike the endocrine glands, secrete their product to the outside, like sweat glands), intestines, blood vessels and external sex organs. This brings us to the autonomic nervous system.

The autonomic nervous system
The autonomic nervous system is responsible for the so-called *involuntary body functions.* Above we already mentioned the exocrine glands, sex organs, blood vessels and intestines (digestion). The healing of diseased body parts is dependent on the autonomic nervous

system. This is composed of two opposing parts: the sympathetic system and the parasympathetic system. Both are responsible for homeostasis ('balance').

The sympathetic nervous system increases the heartbeat when required and keeps digestion in check. The parasympathetic nervous system works in the opposite direction. It lowers the heartbeat when required and stimulates digestion. Like 'yin and yang' or the extensor and flexor muscles in our legs the (antagonistic) sympathetic and parasympathetic nervous systems provide for the proper operation of our body functions.

> *'Because the nervous systems are of paramount importance for optimal functioning of our body nature has provided for optimal protection'*

The above shows that all organs and organ functions are controlled by nervous systems.

Because the systems are of paramount importance for optimal functioning of our body nature has provided for optimal protection. The brain is surrounded by bones (the skull), while the spinal column is surrounded by a complex system of bones, the spinal column. The spinal column is made up of a long row of vertebrae in which the spinal canal is 'locked-in', invulnerable and protected with precision.

The nervous systems are in close contact with one another and one can't function without the other. A defect or disorder of one system implies that the other system too is affected. Under normal circumstances however neither of these systems can be damaged. The skull and spinal column guarantee this. The spinal column provides for the protection of the spinal canal and enables us to move, stand upright and to walk.

Within the spinal cord runs the cerebrospinal fluid. We know it is of great importance for the relaying of nervous impulses, while it also nourishes and purifies the nervous system.

The nerves
From the spinal column the nerves branch of, that's to say 31 pair of nerves, each one composed of billions of fibres. Between the vertebrae there are openings, the 'foramina intervertebralia', which allow the nerve roots to pass through. Besides the spinal cord nerves there are 12 paired cranial nerves, which include the lung/stomach nerve .These cranial nerves lead to the eyes, ears, face and nose and enable us to move our jaws.

Even the smallest irritation of the nervous system may cause a disturbance. The gaps between the vertebrae are the critical spots of the spinal column because that's where the nerve roots pass through. Blocked vertebrae may exert pressure on a nerve. Because of this the normal traffic of nerve impulses is affected (and, so, blocked). The impulses no longer reach the organs and organ functions to a sufficient degree resulting in dysfunction or disease. Optimal health is thus closely linked to the nervous system, while the connection with the spinal column is evident. When blocked vertebrae exert pressure on nerves, all kinds of symptoms may follow. For example, reduced vision or hearing.

5. The locomotor apparatus

*'Because of this process which occurs in a
split second movements pass off
smoothly and harmoniously'*

The locomotor apparatus plays an important role in maintaining optimal health. That's why the chiropractor focusses in particular on the locomotor apparatus. This chapter explains the functioning of the locomotor apparatus.

The locomotor apparatus enables us to move, whereby the bones have a supporting function. The bones are mutually connected by joints. Some joints are more mobile than others. The joint surfaces are covered by cartilage. The mobility of the spinal column is less than that of some of the peripheral joints. The overall mobility of the spinal column is high but the structure of the skeleton and the required functions of the locomotor apparatus imply that the mobility does not have to be the same everywhere. Diametrically opposed to the high mobility of some joints of the limbs is the minimal mobility of the bones of the skull. The joints between the parts of the skull that cover the brain are immovable and are referred to as 'sutures'.

> **The skeleton**
> The locomotor apparatus is very complicated as follows from the fact that it consists of 208 bones, at which 501 muscles are attached.

Main characteristic of the locomotor apparatus

Another characteristic of the locomotor apparatus is the precision of its operation. Via the optic nerve information from the eyes is transmitted to the visual cortex. From there impulses travel to other regions, e.g. to the motor cortex. Next, the correct movements are executed with the required precision and strength. When you lift a very light object you need of course far less force than when you lift a heavy object. Already before the act occurs -the lifting- all the information about this has been processed and passed on. So, the movements are geared to the lifting of the object. Even if it is not known whether the object is light or heavy information about it is transmitted instantly. Receptors (signal receivers) detect and transmit the information (light or heavy) the moment our fingers grip the object. When the object is heavy muscle strength is immediately increased by just the amount needed. Despite the increased muscle power the joints retain their mobility.

In the cerebellum the coordination of locomotion takes place. The cerebellum lies at the bottom of the brain with the posterior (rear) part of the cerebral cortex overlying it and the brainstem (the 'head' of the spinal cord; see chapter 4) in front of it. Both body movements and posture are controlled by the cerebellum. The information of receptors (signal receivers) in the muscles, tendons, joints, eyes, skin and the organ of balance is transmitted to the cerebellum and joined with motor signals from the motor cortex. Next, the integrated signals are transmitted to the cerebral cortex and the spinal cord.

> *'Muscles in resting mode are monitored by the cerebellum and kept in good shape so they can swing into action at any desired moment'*

By means of this process that occurs in a split second movements are executed smoothly and coordinated. Moreover, the cerebellum is responsible for muscle tone. Furthermore, muscles in the resting state are monitored by the cerebellum and kept in good shape so as to enable them to swing into action at the desired moment. After the signals have been processed the nerve impulses from the cerebral cortex travel via the motor nerve to the motor endplate, a structure present at every muscle fibre. At these fine nerve-endings (the endplate) acetylcholine is released, which generates the action potential (electric wave) travelling along the muscle fibre). This action potential is spreads from the motor endplate over the plasma membrane of the muscle. Shortly after a shortening of the muscle fibre occurs, due to the protein filaments from which the muscle is built telescoping. The muscle is then ready to activate a part of the locomotor system. The bones are able to withstand all forces generated. At locations where a greater force is generated the bones are reinforced or supported. Example: the femur demands a stronger bone than elsewhere in the body. That's why the long bone which is in the femur has a thickened shaft in order to enable it to meet the forces involved. The hip bone, too, needs strengthening. In the hip the shaft is supported by tiny *partitions.*

For example: the knee meniscus
As has been stated at the beginning of this chapter the various parts of the skeleton are mutually connected at locations where it is needed. These connections are called joints. There are various kinds of joints: connective tissue joints (or *fixed joints*), joints with limited mobility, the cartilaginous joints and mobile joints, the so-called synovial joints. Synovial fluid (or synovia) is the lubricant in the joint cavity. This is surrounded by the synovial membrane, reinforced by ligaments. Inside the joint cartilaginous structures may be present, for example the meniscus in the knee.

The muscles attach to the bones and make movements possible. But muscles also have a different function. Besides the fact that muscles strengthen the skeleton, muscles also protect the internal organs. They are also important for the proper functioning of the blood circulation. Finally our muscle mass determines the shape of our body. All muscles have their own unique function and the total muscle mass exhibits a huge diversity of shapes. For example the facial muscles express emotions like laughing, crying, surprise.

A very important muscle is the diaphragm or midriff, which is not only required for breathing and stabilising the lower rib during respiration, but which is also involved in moving the torso. The latter also applies to the iliopsoas. The dorsal muscles too have multiple points of attachment to ribs and vertebrae thus enabling the torso to make rotary movements. Muscle activity can occur consciously or unconsciously. There are several types of muscle tissue. Striated muscle can be activated by willpower. Smooth muscle (non-striated) cannot be influenced by our will. These muscles function automatically', autonomously. Heart muscle is special: it consist of autonomic striated muscle.

6. Disturbance of the nervous system

'Each nerve runs from the spinal column to an organ or tissue, so, our nerves can be looked upon as life lines for our organs and tissues'

The chiropractor focuses especially on functional disturbances of the nervous system, or disturbances in the optimal functioning of the nervous system. It may happen that a disturbance manifests itself in the vicinity of spinal cord segments (vertebrae). A displacement of one or more vertebrae may cause a disturbance within the nervous system. This displacement is called a *subluxation*. In most cases that is the location on which the chiropractor focusses during treatment.

Between the vertebrae are openings (foramina intervertebralia) through which the nerve roots pass. Nerve impulses from the brain run through these nerve roots to the organs. When a change occurs in the condition of the spinal column it may happen that these openings become smaller. A nerve can only function properly when it is not interfered with. A slight disturbance along the nerve may already cause irritation and pain. It may even happen that the nerve gets pinched. The flow of nerve impulses is then decreased or cut off. We now know that such a condition can be caused by a so-called *subluxation* ('luxare' is the Latin word for straining or 'dislocation'). Every nerve runs from the spinal column to an organ or tissue, so our nerves can be looked upon as *life lines* for our organs and tissues. Should -theoretically speaking- the nerve impulses fail to reach the organs a life-threatening situation develops. If the flow of nerve impulses decreases - a reduction in supply- disease may ensue.

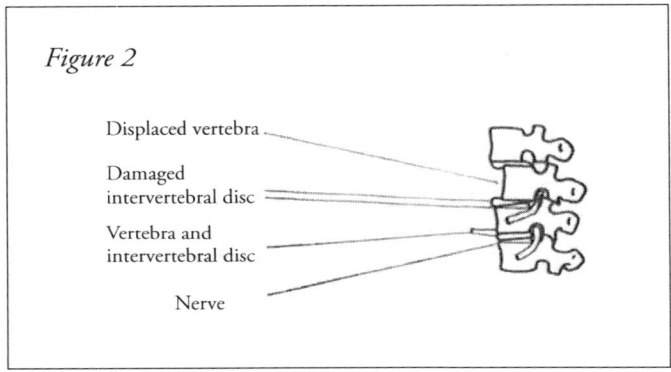

Figure 2

Displaced vertebra
Damaged intervertebral disc
Vertebra and intervertebral disc
Nerve

Figure 2 shows a limitation (disorder) between two vertebrae, a representation of a subluxation. Clearly the nerve is in a wedged position and can no longer perform its task, sending impulses to the organs.

Remember that the spinal column has been assigned a difficult task. The spinal column protects the central nervous system and enables us to walk upright. The spinal column thus carries the whole weight of the upper half of the body including the head. So, we are dealing with tens of kilo's, but the spinal column is up to its task. Between the vertebral bodies the intervertebral discs are located. These are the actual shock absorbers of the spinal column. But those intervertebral discs have to put up with a great deal when the body is in the erect position. They 'suffer' from the constant pressure from the weight of body and head. Also, the body 'turns' constantly, a movement that is also cushioned by the intervertebral discs. These processes may lead to wear and tear. Wrong moves may also result in the fracturing and/or protrusion of intervertebral discs. In the latter case a so-called hernia is present. A disturbance between two vertebrae can be visible, even to the extent that a lay person can observe it with the naked eye. But this damage can be so slight that it cannot be observed and is only tangible to the hands of the doctor or expert chiropractor. Incidentally, not every spinal column blockage needs to damage the nervous system. The situation can be such that the nerves are not affected. But it remains true that a small irritation can lead to damage of the nervous system.

The condition of the body determines the reaction
In conventional medicine the importance of the subluxation is denied. The chiropractor identifies the subluxation is the cause of various symptoms, especially pain in the back or head, neck shoulders, etc. The pain is caused by blocked or irritated nerves, while on the other hand subluxation may result in an increased flow of nerve impulses. This, too, may cause symptoms and pain. The condition of the body determines the response and the intensity of pain. This differs among patients. Further, it should be mentioned that subluxation doesn't always cause symptoms. After all, the vertebrae are always moving during the day as long as the body is moving. Actually subluxations are constantly occurring but a 'motion-disturbance' between two vertebrae is usually automatically corrected. Rarely pain

can be felt fleetingly but usually pain is absent. We thus do not notice anything but nature can be capricious.

As a result of many causes which will be discussed later, it may happen that one or more vertebrae do not automatically return to their designated locations. The vertebra then stays in the wrong position and this subluxation may then cause problems or lead to permanent damage within the spinal column. In the long run the organs will be affected due to a diminished supply of nerve impulses or a the total blockage of nerve impulses. Then the functioning of the nervous system has been affected.

Causes of subluxation
There are many causes of subluxation, so it is hard to identify the most frequent cause. However the list of possible causes may be divided into two categories: the first involving mechanical and psychological causes and the second (less obvious) involving chemical causes. The mechanical courses may occur rather suddenly, the psychological causes less abruptly but still rather quickly, while the chemical causes should be ranged under the heading '*insidious dangers*'. Chemical causes are often not recognized as such .

Mechanical causes
Mechanical causes occur as a result of performing wrong acts or incidents by which in a split second something goes wrong in the spinal column. Mostly the mechanical causes are obvious. But what kind of things can go wrong?

> **Causes of displaced vertebrae**
> - Mechanical causes
> - Psychological causes
> - Chemical causes

Everyone has sometimes had the experience that after having stooped one feels something *snap* in the back. Then you have difficulty straightening yourself and you feel intense pain in your back or legs. Such a situation represents the best illustration of a subluxation. Here the 'motion-disturbance' between two vertebrae has not corrected itself in a natural way. Sometimes the pain immediately disappears when standing upright: the vertebra has slipped back to its proper position in the spinal column. But sometimes the pain lasts longer, for example a couple of days, and eventually the vertebra returns to the position where it belongs. But the pain can also persist and then the subluxation becomes 'permanent': the vertebra is permanently irritated. But the pain may also disappear while the disturbance remains. This is the most dangerous situation. For you think everything is back to normal but this is not the case. Pain can appear later, a couple of weeks later, but even years later! In that case the nerve is wedged but the total supply of nerve impulses is not (yet) blocked. So, sometimes pain can come on long after the incident so that one no longer remembers the reason. The same (often sudden) situation can of course also occur during heavy physical exertion. When one lifts a heavy object subluxation can suddenly occur.

> *'Sometimes pain can come on long after the incident so that one no longer remembers the reason'*

It can also happen while chopping wood or in the case of a garage mechanic constantly stooping over the engine or someone who during his job has to perform other *difficult* movements. It can happen while working in the house or garden. But people with a strenuous physical job are constantly exposed to the risk of subluxation. This also holds true for housewives who have to stoop, kneel, stretch a lot, etc. Especially stretching (e.g. taking off the curtains) can lead to subluxation. In summary: a subluxation can quickly develop in anyone who often stoops or kneels or makes body movements for which the spinal column is not always designed. From this it follows that people who tend to overtax their body run a greater risk of subluxation due to a mechanical cause than people with a sedentary profession. Still the latter group is also at risk. In the office much can go wrong, if only sitting on poor office chair, reaching for a dossier above your head or frequently having to stoop for dossiers filed away too low. People who drive a lot run a risk. We often sit in seats unsuited for our spinal column. Getting in or out of the car, carrying heavy briefcases (think of salesmen) can cause a subluxation. Shop workers are also at risk. But sitting on poorly designed seats, both at home and/or in the car can result in a subluxation which is sometimes neither visible nor palpable. These people run the risk of an insidious subluxation with pain developing much later, often, as mentioned, after years. We often sit (or, better:

sprawl) in the evening on uncomfortable settees. That too is not conducive to a healthy back.

Another possible cause of a direct luxation is of course falling, at home, at work or in the street. Then, too, something may happen that is immediately palpable. But here too the symptoms may develop only much later, sometimes years later! A car accident can of course cause instant problems. Being struck by another car from behind can cause whiplash. The neck receives a vicious rap which can cause pain now or later. Years later neck pain, headache, listlessness and depression may result from such a collision.

Psychic causes
It is scientifically well-established that emotions too can have pathological consequences. Negative emotions like anxiety, depression, anger, grief, jalousie, resentment, etc. may thus cause physical symptoms. The resulting symptoms are then called psychosomatic disorders. Depression can cause tense muscles, especially around the spinal column. If the depression lasts longer the abnormal muscles tension may become chronic. This can lead to subluxations. In chapters 4 and 5 we explained the interaction between the spinal column and muscles. When the back muscles are constantly tense vertebrae can be chronically put under strain and at a certain moment be permanently pulled from their correct position. Again a common cause of subluxation.

Sometimes the consequences are not immediately apparent, but occasionally they are (see chapter 13, *Stress and chiropractic*). When it concerns emotions and stress not directly pointing at the spinal column they are often not recognized as a possible cause of subluxation. When one is constantly under stress one is nervous and irritated. Tense muscles can be the direct consequence of this. Subconsciously the muscles are then tensed in an abnormal way. So, (almost) every movement becomes an unnatural movement and relaxed muscles are a thing of the past. Here the chiropractor can of course do little about the causes. Where grief or other problems are the cause of nervous exhaustion the individual needs to solve these him- or herself, or with the help of a psychologist. The chiropractor will certainly offer advice but cannot really tackle the root problem. It should be clear that solving emotional problems is of essential importance for physical health. Just correcting the subluxation will not lead to a permanent (re) solution of the physical problems.

> '*Solving emotional problems is of essential importance for physical health*'

For, after all, we're taking for granted that a cure doesn't only tackle the symptoms but eliminates the cause just as well. It wouldn't be an exaggeration to say that solving the cause is many times more important than solving the symptom, the subluxation. It should be clear that especially negative emotions are destructive for good health, for example egoism, resentment, bottled up hate, jalousie and perverted exercise of power. Positive emotions such as tolerance, acceptance, love, harmony and empathy on the contrary exert a healing effect. These thoughts and emotions can be so strong that just by a change to positive emotions subluxations and symptoms can be resolved.

Chemical causes
Chemical factor may serve as possible causes of subluxation: insidious causes as subluxation develops only after years of exposure. Which chemical factors may be involved?

Without being conscious of it we are constantly exposed to 'attacks from outside', such as air pollution from factories, exhaust fumes from cars, etc. But also chemical pollution of the body from polluted food, that is food with colourings, flavourings and artificial odours. Drinks too contain artificial substances to fortify the taste or to give the drink a 'nice colour'. The meat we buy at the butcher's is not always originally really as red. But since it has been drummed into us that good meat should be red the butcher adds some colour to the meat, again a chemical substance.

Chemical substances or hormones may have been administered to the animal to accelerate its growth. The products of the greengrocer have probably been treated with chemicals as well in order to protect these against insects or to accelerate their growth. Our alcoholic drinks contain chemicals too, while smoking seriously pollutes our bodies. Moreover we use drugs like sleeping pills and tranquilizers, another source of pollution.

In summary: every year we consume pounds of chemicals, breathe polluted air or pollute our body in other ways. This pollution thus causes *chemical subluxation*. That means that the body responds to pollution. The body resists foreign substances and protests against them. Though it is an insidious hazard since the consequences of pollution only become gradually manifest, subluxation can nonetheless be its direct result. We should remain aware of it.

Other causes
This long list of possible causes of a displaced position of a vertebra cannot be complete. Numerous other causes may underlie it. For example sport. Sportsters are constantly exposed to dangers: wrong moves, little accidents, excessive effort, etc. (see chapter 9, *Sport and chiropractic)*. Pregnancy can cause spinal column problems, as does child birth, both for mother and child. Also the child as toddler or older is at risk. The child plays and romps, falls and it climbs and is thus exposed to risks possibly leading to subluxation and symptoms. Especially for children, toddlers included, chiropractic can be effective.

Though the regular physician may often overlook the subluxation, the chiropractor focusses on the aforementioned and other symptoms and their possible causes. We should not overlook the spinal column. The chiropractor certainly won't!

7. To the chiropractor

> *'A pity that the chiropractor still sees patients who for instance have been suffering from backache for years or from migraine for half their lives'*

It still happens that people are ignorant about chiropractic and thus have no idea what a chiropractor does and how to find him. Patients consult a chiropractor only after having learnt about chiropractic from colleagues, friends or relatives who have been treated or are being treated by a chiropractor. Fortunately, the familiarity and popularity of chiropractic is on the rise and patients find their way through articles, talks, the internet or TV programs. An increasing number of people are looking for alternative ways aimed at health and healing.

People are fed up with painkillers, sleeping pills and other drugs. Unfortunately far too few patients are being referred to the chiropractor by a family doctor, specialist or therapist. But the number of referrals is on the rise.

Still it is a pity that the chiropractor still sees patients who have been - for example - suffering from backache for fifteen or twenty years or from migraine for half their lives. Patients who could have been helped much earlier but who were ignorant about the existence of chiropractic. And don't forget: in schools and universities chiropractic and other *alternative treatments* are completely ignored. Since the general knowledge about chiropractic is so limited this chapter will explain how the first contacts are made, from the health insurer to the examination by the chiropractor.

Step by step we'll now follow the patient from the waiting room onward.

In the waiting room
In the waiting room of the chiropractor generally few patients will be found. The chiropractor can determine rather precisely how much time will be needed for each patient. The first visit will last about an hour, further treatments depending on the circumstances will require 20 - 30 minutes. So nobody has to wait longer than required and each patient is received at the time of the appointment.

*'The atmosphere in the waiting room is relaxed.
A relief for both adults and children'*

One rarely meets complaining patients in the waiting room or patients who look ill, as happens so often in the waiting room of family doctors and specialists. Usually the waiting patients have already had a number of treatments with improvement of their situation. No coughing and sneezing children, no complaining about illnesses, no anxious patients, no fearful children… There is also no fear of injections or new drugs; there is no fear because one does not know what disorder one is suffering from, or fear of referral to a specialist or hospital… In short, a relaxed atmosphere will be found in the waiting room of the chiropractor. A relief for both adults and children.

Case history and discussion
Anyone entering the waiting room will feel relaxed. The first thing one notices is the absence of the penetrating antiseptic smell one often finds in the waiting rooms of doctors and hospitals.

The first conversation with the patient will take at least half an hour and the physical examination another thirty minutes. So, the patient gets plenty of attention, very different from a visit to the family doctor, which lasts ten minutes at the most, after which one is ushered out with a prescription in hand.

During the talk the chiropractor goes into a lot of questions. Of course he needs to know the symptoms but the talk is also meant to find out the cause of the symptoms. First the chiropractor may want to know the duration of the symptoms and will next go into the case history and the patient's lifestyle (!). This is done to establish how the symptoms might have arisen.

The chiropractor will ask e.g. the following questions:

- Have you ever been involved in an accident?
- Have you ever had a bad fall?
- How are the working conditions?
- Do you do any heavy work?

- What is the nature of this (heavy) work?
- Do you often have to stoop or rotate the body?
- Do you often have to lift heavy objects?
- Do you have hobbies requiring heavy physical exertion?
- Do you practise a sport? Is it a strenuous sport?
- Have you ever undergone surgery?
- Have you been treated for symptoms by your family doctor or specialist? If affirmative, what kind of treatment did you receive?
- How about medicines, narcotics, alcohol?
- Do you consume more alcohol than two drinks daily?
- What kind of food do you usually eat?
- Are there any problems at home or at your work?
- Do you live under a lot of stress?
- How do you sleep and how do you sit at home in chairs or on the couch?

The answers to these questions provide the chiropractor with a clear picture about the patient. On the basis of this picture and the physical examination a diagnosis will be made. Then the chiropractor will explain his plan of action and its limitations. Perhaps he may show you a model of the spinal column as an *illustration* of what might have happened to the vertebrae.

Further the chiropractor may show with the aid of illustrations how the nervous system works. He will also tell you about the physical examination and about the nature of the treatment should it be required. What happens during the treatment and how long it will take: he/she will also give you an estimate about the chance of success. The chiropractor will tell you the total costs of the treatments and advices, so it will not come as a surprise. The advices are about exercises the patient can perform at home, sleeping on the right matrass, healthy nutrition, better method of working, both at home and in the workplace, etc.

It should be clear that the chiropractor devotes plenty of time to establish a diagnosis, how the symptoms developed and can be dealt with and especially to make clear to the patient which path will probably lead to improvement of the situation. After his first visit the patient will have learnt a good deal about the functioning of the human body in general and his/her own in particular.

The physical examination
The extensive talk is followed by the physical examination. The patient is asked to remove the shirt or the blouse and lies down on a specially constructed couch. This couch is about two meters long and has a recess for the head. The patient is asked to lie on his stomach. Without the recess the head would be turned sideways resulting in a rotation of the neck, both for the therapist and the patient a most undesirable position. The first part of the examination is formed by *palpations*.

There are two different forms of palpations. The first is called *'static palpations'*. The chiropractor feels the spinal column and, directed by the patient's response, identifies sensitive or painful locations along the spinal column and any tensed up muscles.

Whether displaced vertebrae are visible or palpable....
The chiropractor also feels each vertebra separately. He tries to establish if it is indeed a matter of a displaced vertebra. As stated before it is possible that it may be visible by the unaided eye, but in most cases this will not be the case. An expert chiropractor will certainly feel the displaced vertebra.

The second type of palpations is called '*motion palpations*'.

The patient is asked to stand up and to bend forwards and backwards, to the left and to the right. He/she will now be palpated in different positions and in this situation it will be assessed whether displaced vertebrae are visible or palpable. It is possible that now a movement disturbance becomes manifest (visible and/or palpable) in a certain position of the body, while another position doesn't manifest the subluxation. That's why the expression 'motion palpations'. Experience tells us that a subluxation is often accompanied by a difference in leg length. This difference can be relatively large, e.g. one centimetre, but it can also be a matter of only a few millimetres.

If a subluxation is neither visible nor palpable then the difference in leg length may (!) indicate the presence of a subluxation. Anyway, the difference in leg length will be corrected after treatment. That's why the leg length is measured during diagnosis and again after a few sessions. If after a certain moment the difference in leg length has disappeared it strengthens the assumption that the subluxation has been removed. Of course this is just one method to establish the diagnosis.

> '*The chiropractor can take X-ray pictures of the whole spinal column, the skull, and of parts of the spinal column*'

The chiropractor inspects the patient in *his totality*, that is, while at rest and in motion as well as in different positions. It may happen that one shoulder is a bit lower than the other. That too can be indicative of a subluxation. It may be mentioned in passing that when the chiropractor concludes on the basis of his observations that the posture of the patient is poor the patient will be told about this. Advice for improvement will be given, including exercises and posture correction.

When the examination suggests a disturbance of the nervous system or a subluxation then the chiropractor may take one or more X-ray pictures. The X-ray picture too offers additional evidence of a possible subluxation. The chiropractor may take pictures of the whole spinal column, the skull, and of parts of the spinal column. The X-ray picture doesn't only serve as confirmation of a subluxation, but also whether there are '*underlying diseases*' and thus circumstances that prohibit performing the 'manipulations'. The X-ray picture offers a clearer picture of the general physical condition and thus serves a number of 'purposes'. It will not be possible to identify the subluxation from the picture in all cases, but then other diagnostic methods may achieve this. In any case the chiropractor knows, after this exhaustive examination, what is expected of him and he will be able to gear these findings to a treatment programme.

When the subluxation has been amply established the examination will be completed. It may however happen that the chiropractor utilizes a supplementary diagnosis. For example the chiropractor may measure muscle strength at both sides of the body. If differences are found this may serve as another clue.

To the chiropractor

* Referral required? No
* Is the treatment reimbursed? Yes, in most cases
* At the chiropractor:
  - Conversation chiropractor-patient
  - Medical history
  - Symptoms
* Physical examination:
  - Static palpations
  - Motion palpations
  - Possibly X-ray pictures
  - Additional diagnostics
* Treatment scheme:
  - Number of visits
  - Compliance with advice with regard to food, exercise, posture, etc.

Much depends on the condition of the patient
It should be noted that the diagnosis is not always carried out in the way described above. Much depends on the condition of the patient and the views of the chiropractor in question. Not every chiropractor will measure temperature differences on both sides of the spinal column. Further, he made not consider the taking of X-ray pictures necessary. It may be that the chiropractor considers the situation sufficiently evident, or that he finds the X-ray radiation objectionable (see chapter 16. *Schools within chiropractic*). Also, the patient himself made object against the taking of X-ray pictures. We're here dealing with a very low dose of radiation that is considered absolutely harmless.

If the diagnosis shows that the patient does not qualify for a chiropractic treatment the chiropractor will refer the patient to a doctor. The chiropractor will never treat a patient if it is not clear that the treatment may be successful. In special cases the chiropractor will contact another therapist, family doctor or specialist, of course in close consultation with the patient. If a disturbance is present justifying chiropractic treatment the chiropractor will of course proceed to action.

8. The treatment

'A symptom may be present for a week but sometimes for years or dozens of years. It is evident that in the latter case more treatment sessions will be needed'

The examination completed, the chiropractor will tell the patient what will be done to help the patient as quickly as possible. Sometimes the chiropractor can determine in advance how many sessions will be needed. In most cases this will not be possible because the number of treatments depends on a number of factors. To name a few: age, the nature and severity of the symptom, the duration of the symptom, etc. A symptom may be present for a week or sometimes for years or dozens of years. It is evident that in the latter case more treatment sessions will be needed. How many is hard to tell as the chiropractor doesn't yet know how the body will respond to the treatment. Sometimes the body already to the first treatment, sometimes only after tree or for sessions. Anyway, generally the number of sessions does not exceed ten.

The pressure can be light, sometimes heavier
The procedure is as follows. The patient lies on his stomach on the table. The chiropractor now knows which vertebrae are irritated and thus require corrective action. The chiropractor starts with exerting a (usually) light pressure on the blocked spinal cord

segments (vertebrae) and possibly also on other vertebrae. This will be done in different ways. First, when the patient lies on his /her stomach. But the patient must now and again assume a different lying position, sometimes with an arm above the head, sometimes on the left side, sometimes on the right. In all these positions the chiropractor exerts pressure on the vertebrae, especially on the affected or irritated vertebrae that have caused the functional disturbance within the nervous system. The pressure can be light, sometimes heavier. Now and again a cracking sound may be heard, a click. This is caused by a sudden energy transfer within the joint.

Without the patient noticing because of his position(s) the chiropractor performs various actions. A constant pressure lasting seconds may be followed by a quick push against one of the vertebrae. Both during and after the treatment the chiropractor constantly observes the body's position.

The chiropractor treats and observes the patient also in the vertical position. The shoulders too receive attention in order to correct positional asymmetry.

No pain
The treatment at the chiropractor is painless, although the pressure exerted on the vertebrae may sometimes be felt, or rarely the patient may start visibly from a sudden correction. To repeat: pain or irritation are absent. During the treatment the chiropractor may place the patient on a stool. He will then sit behind the patient and performs again the actions as described

above or observes the body's position, now while the patient is sitting. The action intended to correct displaced vertebrae is called an *'adjustment'*.

The response to adjustments
As we know subluxation is the result of blocked vertebrae, or a 'motion-disturbance' between two vertebrae by which nerves might have been wedged. As a result the rate of nerves impulses diminishes or stops altogether, this while the organs require it, depend on it. When the chiropractor manipulates the vertebrae the blockade can sometimes be lifted within one or two treatments. As a result the nerve impulses can suddenly flow freely. Little wonder that the wedged nerve will get a bit of a *fright*. For the blockade may be the cause of the impulse supply having been restricted for years. Now, since the nerve has 'regained its freedom' the *adjustment* may have released an enormous supply of nerve impulses, signals penetrating deep into the nervous system, from one moment to the other. This may result in a stiff neck or tingling in the head. Further other chemical reactions occur in the body. In many parts of the body blood flow may improve while other body fluids (e.g. lymph fluid) will circulate more freely again. The blood sugar content may suddenly rise.

> *'As a result the nerve impulses can suddenly flow freely. Little wonder that the wedged nerve will get a bit of a fright'*

Especially after the first treatment the body can react in different ways. Some patients will feel much better as a result of these sudden reactions, even feeling very energetic. But it may also be that one feels heavy and sleepy. Or there may be a headache or a slight sense of being unwell. Tiredness too may be present after the first treatment. These are all very normal and predictable reactions of the body. Apart from the sudden free flow of nerve impulses the muscles too will again function normally after having been wedged in for a long time. The body has to cope with all this because it had become used to the situation and had neglected many tasks that it now resumes immediately. We have to realize that each body is unique and that we cannot predict how it will react to a new situation. One body may feel better right away, the other may feel a bit worse for a little while. But every reaction is normal and a less pleasant reaction will soon disappear. The body will feel grateful for the improved condition and the patient soon feels better, usually within hours after treatment.

The reaction to the treatment of the same symptom among several patients may differ. In some patients the pain in the back or in the head will have disappeared after only one treatment. In others a series of treatments will be required to bring relieve. As we have seen a disturbance may have been present for years. It is obvious that this disturbance cannot always be cured in one treatment.

The human body is difficult to fathom
Whatever reaction the body displays, there is no risk in the hands of an expert chiropractor. When it con-

cerns a very clear symptom, one that is directly related to the position of the spinal column and the 'motion-disturbance' between two vertebrae, then it rarely happens that no improvement is seen after a number of treatments. The chiropractor can almost guarantee that the symptom obviously caused by a subluxation will improve after treatment. *Almost*, since the human body is difficult to fathom. But in the rare cases that no improvement occurs the chiropractor will not continue forever with the treatments. He/she will not hesitate to tell you that the symptom does not respond to the treatment and in consultation with the patient another solution will be sought, for example referral to another therapist or doctor. In any case symptoms like backache, pain in the neck or shoulders, pain in the joints, almost always will respond rather quickly to a treatment, as well as symptoms due to irritation of the nervous system.

The standard scheme is one session a week. In a rare case treatment is started with two sessions weekly, followed by once a week. In general it can be stated that a patient needs six to eight treatments, sometimes more, sometimes less.

The Chiropractor is not a miracle doctor
Perhaps one may think that the chiropractor should be regarded as a kind of *miracle doctor*. But *miracle doctors* don't exist. But the chiropractor is a therapist who can resolve many symptoms and he accomplishes this with what nature has given us: the body's ability to cope with symptoms.

The chiropractor assists dormant nature in arousing the nervous system. The inborn capacity of every living being to cope with symptoms is awakened by the treatments. But the fact remains that the human body is one of the most complex *machines* one can imagine and that means that no doctor or therapist exists who can resolve everything. Cancer is a case in point. Not enough is known about the development of cancer. Chiropractors will definitely not claim they can be of any help against serious diseases like cancer or multiple sclerosis. The chiropractor can also do little against bacterial or viral infections.

The chiropractor will point this out to the patient. In case the chiropractor discovers a serious disease the patient will be referred to his family doctor.

After the treatment
Let us assume the chiropractic treatment has been successful. What then? Opinions differ. Some say it is pointless to visit the chiropractor periodically for examination and possible treatment. Although the subluxation may develop from one moment to the next this '*movement*' holds that it is early enough to consult the chiropractor when new symptoms arise. We don't agree with this opinion because the subluxation presents a dormant risk. The subluxation can occur 'without warning' and only many years later symptoms may become manifest that are more severe than when the subluxation had been identified and treated earlier. The nervous system is complex and one kind of damage may lead to further damage somewhere else in the body.

We thus agree with the movement that posits that it makes sense to visit the chiropractor periodically for a check-up. So, even if there are no symptoms; it exerts a preventive action and is highly advisable for patients who have been relieved of their symptoms.

One could visit the chiropractor, say, twice a year for a check-up. Physical problems can thus be prevented and the costs are low.

This check-up is the more important for the so-called high-risk group. This includes people with a strenuous physical job (housewives included!), children and older people. In most cases the chiropractor will advise the patient on how to prevent symptoms. So, it concerns healthier eating habits, exercises, a better life-style or changes in living conditions, both at home and at work (better matrass, different chairs, etc.). Another advice should be added: live a life of total awareness and think about all the things that may happen. Just by being more aware a lot of physical problems can be prevented.

NB: In view of the different movements in chiropractic (chapter 16) the way of thinking and treatment methods may differ among chiropractors.

9. Sport and chiropractic

'Despite the benefits of sport various symptoms may develop. Sportsmen and sportswomen are constantly exposed to the risk of injuries'

Various organs and body functions are taxed by sport: the vertebrae, the muscles, the joints, heart and lungs. Of course sport is good for you because by using your muscles and taxing your heart and lungs you improve your physical fitness, while this change from the daily routine like work, watching TV and the computer screen may be regarded as an excellent form of mental relaxation.

Going in for sport offers both physical and mental benefits. However this does not hold for strenuous sporting achievements. Because of this the organs may in many cases be overtaxed.

A too abrupt increase of physical activity, especially in certain forms of contest may cause problems. Despite the benefits of sport various symptoms may develop. Sportsmen/sportswomen are constantly exposed to the risk of injuries. Often these injuries are of a general nature, usually innocuous and easy to prevent by a proper *warming up* and well supervised training.

In the earlier chapters it was shown that many apparently innocent looking injuries (bumping, falling, etc.) later can lead to symptoms of a more serious nature. A regular check-up by a chiropractor can prevent a lot of trouble while the chiropractor is also the right therapist to treat the more serious injuries. Remember, the chiropractor is specialized in treating the spinal column, muscles and joints and it is these systems that are taxed in sports and sustain injuries.

Common injuries
Both individual sports and team sports carry risks. Some injuries are innocuous and disappear spontaneously, while other injuries may carry the risk of permanent damage. Damage that in most cases is not directly visible but which may cause problems at an older age. Every sportsman/sportswoman is familiar with these injuries which are almost the order of the day: strained muscles, muscle fatigue, cramps, fissures in the cartilage, damage to tendons, bumps, bruises, concussions and bone fractures. Briefly we'll discuss some of these common sport-related injuries that can be addressed by the chiropractor.

Neck injuries
Neck injuries occur especially during rough sports like rugby, a sport that puts great stress on the body. Rugby clashes may result in neck damage. In archers, too, straining the neck is a common complaint. Riders, beginners as well as experienced ones, may suffer falls which often cause neck injuries.

Shoulder injuries
Shoulder dislocation and shoulder sprain are often found in sports like rugby (heavy stress on the

shoulders), archery, skeet-shooting, various field games (like hockey), golf, judo, swimming, cricket, bowling and 'martial arts'.

Arm injuries
Arm injuries often occur in martial arts, including boxing, wrestling and again rugby.

Elbow injuries
Elbow joint injuries are often seen in golfers and tennis players.

Wrists
Pain in the wrists is often seen in sports like tennis, judo, volleyball, badminton, squash and weight lifting.

Hands and feet
Injuries to fingers and hands, bone fractures end dislocations are often seen in boxing and other martial arts, but also in skating, roller-skating, cricket and rugby.

Back injuries
There are few sports that do not carry the risk of back injuries. Spinal column injurie especially occur in sports with intense physical aggression, for example soccer, rugby, martial arts but also (other) ball games, weight lifting, riding, playing skittles or bowling, tennis and even jogging.

Tail bone
Tail bone problems often occur in riding. Especially at jumping the rider may land badly in the saddle.

Abdominal muscles
Especially in weightlifting subjective symptoms about abdominal muscles are frequently heard.

Knee
In most sports heavy demand is made on the knee joint. Symptoms like sprain of knee joints, muscle and tendon inflammation, bursitis often occur in rugby, soccer, golf, skiing, skating, roller-skating, cycling and jogging.

Ankles
Ankle sprains and Achilles tendon inflammation are often seen in tennis, badminton, skiing, athletics, soccer and other field sports and jogging.

Feet and toes
Inflammation of the sole and fractures of the toes are seen in field sports and jogging.

Summary of common sport injuries

* Abdominal muscles symptoms
* Achilles tendon inflammation
* Arm injuries
* Back symptoms
* Bone fractures
* Bursitis
* Cartilage fissures
* Concussion
* Cramped muscles
* Dislocations
* Elbow symptoms
* Fatigued muscles
* Fractures
* Ligament damage
* Neck injuries (strain)
* Scratches
* Shoulder dislocation
* Shoulder strain
* Sole inflammation.
* Sprain-ankle
* Sprain-knee
* Swellings
* Tail bone problems
* Tendon damage
* Tendon inflammation
* Wrists pain

How to prevent sport injuries

When one looks at the list of possible injuries one might be tempted to conclude that the practice of sport is a risky business. This is definitely not the case. Sport can certainly promote health. But sport may involve risks if one goes about it rashly. Sport injuries are only too often the direct result of a poor training programme, irregular training, hurried training to obtain quick results, or a training not sufficiently attuned to the sport in question. Further one should ask oneself what one wishes to achieve with sport. One may aim for greater endurance, for improved efficiency or for improved muscle strength. Fine objectives, but if you aim at a semi-professional level you would be well advised to hire a professional trainer.

Training

A good trainer won't rush you into achieving great results without taking into account the specific circumstances of the individual. Age is taken into account, as well as the medical history (old injuries?) and other factors health-related factors. For that matter the serious sportsman himself should take these factors into account. If pain occurs during training or if straining or sprain is present then the trainer should be told immediately. No-one but the sportsman himself can better indicate what happens to his body during exercises.

> *'No-one but the sportsman himself can better indicate what happens to his body during exercises'*

Further, most sports require special clothing, shoes, gloves, sport bra's, glasses, etc. Also special apparatus is often used like in health clubs. For example dumbbells and other weight-lifting gear and gear to increase muscle strength. One should heed the advice of the trainer while using this equipment. Incorrect use may also result in injuries.

Minor and serious injuries
Minor injuries can be treated by the sportsman or – woman him/herself. For example bruises, bumps, scratches, blisters. When serious injuries occur which are related to muscles, joints, ligaments or the back then it is advisable to consult a chiropractor. The chiropractor can then decide whether the injury can be treated by the sportsman/sportswomen himself/herself or whether it qualifies for chiropractic treatment. In some cases a compression or an exercise will be sufficient. In other cases the sometimes invisible damage can only be corrected by chiropractic treatment.

The chiropractic treatment
Generally the treatment can start immediately when you consult the chiropractor at an early stage. In the USA and the UK top sportsmen are continuously being looked after by a chiropractor or are under chiropractic supervision.

10. Children and chiropractic

'Backache is supposed to happen to the elderly, but surely not to children....'

Symptoms of the spinal column often turn out to have originated in early youth. This is often ignored. Backache is supposed to happen to the elderly, but surely not to children ... A child plays and horses about, looks healthy and sound, eats well and behaves normally. Still, something could happen or has happened that will cause problems later in life.

Disturbances of the spinal vertebra are invisible and cannot be felt. Besides, the child does not complain easily and not at all when the pain after a fall or a jolt disappears spontaneously. Still falls can be the cause of permanent damage. Especially with regard to children the saying holds, 'an ounce of prevention is worth a pound of cure'. The chiropractor can make a diagnosis and make corrections at an early stage so the child will not be troubled in his further development by (sometimes still) minor disturbances. A good example is the fairly common *curvature of the spine*. But apart from this there are further risks.

As has been mentioned before the spinal column is of great importance for the proper functioning of the body and for health in general. The intervertebral discs play an important role as shock absorbers that cushion blows and heavily taxed in youth. Despite the protection by bones and these shock absorbers much can happen to a toddler, child or young adult.

Apparently harmless incidents
Don't forget that apparently harmless incidents do occur. For example a baby may fall off the table while mom is changing his nappy. Over-enthusiastic parents, brothers or sisters may drop a baby, while something can go frightfully wrong while playfully throwing the little kid into the air. While learning to walk the child falls many times against furniture or on the floor and also playing with dogs or other children can result in jolts and thrusts.

Every parent knows the result: crying binges, knee injuries and bruises. It shows the child is temporarily in pain. Pain that is quickly soothed by father or mother and the child forgets the incident just as fast. Still, it cannot be excluded that the vertebra is unable to fully deal with this process of constant jolts and vibrations. Later in life problems may arise (backache, headache, etc.) which have their roots in early childhood.

Jolts and thrusts in pre-school age is just part of the picture. As the child grows older it learns to ride a bike, ride a horse perhaps the child goes in for skating, roller-skating, soccer, roller blading, hockey, skiing or sports involving intense physical aggression. In puberty the child is perhaps interested in cross-country cycling, cycling or mopeds where jolts and falls are the order of the day. In only a few cases it is immediately clear that something has gone wrong. But in most cases the pain disappears and it seems that no damage has been done. Often pain is regarded as normal. But this is only true of *growth pains* that are supposed to be part of growing up. In reality these pains can be the result of vertebra problems.

> 'Still it cannot be ruled out that the vertebra is
> unable to fully deal with this
> process of constant jolts and vibration'

The long list of possible causes is not complete. Just like adults children (and especially children) can get habituated to a poor posture. They too can subconsciously suffer from poor 'work conditions'. Perhaps they sleep on poor beds and slouch on soft couches for hours watching TV or playing video games. School desks that are too low for tall kids may also be a factor. During many hours kids are working bending forward in their seat. The developing spinal column doesn't get the needed support.

The back of a child is very flexible and developing constantly. Obviously the young spinal column needs a good school desk, a good desk, a good matrass and a good chair for watching TV. This will promote a good posture. Alas, the reality is different…..

Chiropractic holds that children with spinal column problems can quickly be helped by correction of the spine and the *adjustments* discussed earlier: so, applying a dosed mechanical impulse carried out with the hands or with the aid of instruments. The treatment is painless. The chiropractor corrects the position of the vertebrae, influences the joints positively and increases the body's mobility.

When to visit a chiropractor with your child?
In view of all the risks during early childhood and later it is advisable to regularly visit the chiropractor with your child for a check-up and, if required, for preventive treatment. There is much at stake with regard to the child's health later in life. Parents tend to believe that harmless crying, scrapes and bumps are inconsequential. In most cases this is true. Bumps and scrapes disappear as does the pain. But in a rare case the foundation is laid for unpleasant consequences. Curvature of the spine is one of them, a defect that may involve neurological consequences. The chiropractor identifies the symptoms, makes the diagnosis and is able to treat virtually any disturbance of the spinal column. It is important that he/she is able to explain clearly and simply what has gone wrong and how the disturbance can be corrected.

The treatment
Before reaching the diagnosis the chiropractor will first look closely at the child's medical history. Has the child ever been ill, or there any relevant living conditions that might have led to problems? The physical examination focuses in particular on the spinal column and coccyx. Posture too is examined and the vertebrae are palpated. If the nervous system is irritated it can be detected is this way. The X-ray machine

will only be used when necessary. If the examination shows that a chiropractic treatment is indicated, the chiropractor will manipulate the vertebrae or apply a correction by means of the adjustments discussed above. The treatments are painless and the number of treatments depends on the severity of the disturbance.

Regular check-ups contribute to the health of the child. Problems at a later age are, as mentioned, thus prevented. A third of the population suffers occasionally or continuously from backache. With extra care during childhood much of this pain might have been prevented. The chiropractor can play an important role in that.

11. Pregnancy and chiropractic

*'A delivery under analgesics or a delivery via
Caesarian may cause harm to the child'*

Not only during youth a lot can go wrong with the child: even in the pre-natal stage a lot can happen, for example, if the physical condition of the pregnant woman leaves much to be desired. Also the expectant mother may have had a nasty fall at home or outside or may have suffered an accident. Furthermore the child may be injured as a result of a difficult delivery, like a delivery with the aid of instruments.

During a protected delivery the mother is physically taxed to the limit. A delivery under analgesics or a delivery via Caesarian may cause harm to the child. Even at a normal smooth going delivery injuries can happen. For example in the final stage of the delivery when the baby is having a hard time as the head or neck is being pulled hard. But even serious injuries are often not directly visible and this also holds for injuries to vertebrae or the skull.

Negative effects on the vertebra of the baby
Especially injuries during delivery may lead to physiological dysfunction. The exceptional forces exerted by instruments during delivery can have negative effects on the baby's spine. Migraine or headache occurring

much later is rarely traced to childbirth events. Still it can happen that this is the cause of later symptoms.

It goes without saying that it is assumed that the expectant mother takes good care of herself and that the doctors assisting the delivery are competent. Since it is possible that the child, despite all possible precautions before or during delivery, may have sustained injuries the parents would be well advised to consult a chiropractor for a check-up. He/she will be able to assess any possible damage and prevent further trouble by an effective treatment at this early stage in the life of the child.

12. Elderly people and chiropractic

*'Chiropractic doesn't simply accept ailments
and pains that are supposed to
be caused by old age'*

Ever since childhood it has been drummed into us that old age is simply associated with 'the ailments of old age'. In other words, symptoms and ailments must be accepted as your lot when you are old: there is nothing you can do about it. That's why many older people just simply accept having to live with pain and with ailments and symptoms.

Even the doctor tells the patient that his/her symptoms are related to age and so the elderly patient leaves the doctor's office with a prescription for a synthetic drug, another addition to the medicine chest. But the big question is, 'can really nothing be done about these so-called ailments of old age?'

Chiropractic doesn't resign itself to ailments and pains supposedly caused by age. The chiropractor has shown himself to be able to treat many of these symptoms effectively. Even when there is no question of a cure at least pain reduction can be achieved, joints can be made more flexible and stiffness lessened.

The elderly person is especially bothered by symptoms relating to the spinal column and the joints. Bones of older people can become more brittle and joints stiffer and so less flexible, the chiropractor 's main field of interest. He examines the condition of the bones and joints, assesses the medical history and is thus able to offer a treatment program benefiting many elderly people.

Aching joints
After examining patients with painful joints the diagnosis usually is: arthritis. However, arthritis is but an umbrella term for various conditions. It may concern a joint inflammation caused by rheumatic conditions. The inflammation may also have been caused by an injury or an infection. The cause of the joint inflammation is of paramount importance. When the cause is known the treatment can be tailored to it. Needless to say that an acute infection will not be treated by a chiropractor. This should be left to the family doctor or the specialist. But often after the inflammation has been cured the pain persists. This pain may be successfully treated by the chiropractor. He/she can make sure that the pain disappears or is greatly reduced.

Let's take arthritis of the hip joint as an example, a common complaint in the elderly. Hip replacement operations can do a lot of good, but generally the waiting lists are long. During the waiting period the movement of the spinal vertebrae, the pelvis and the affected hip can be stimulated. As a result the pain is reduced considerably and the freedom of movement is increased.

Frozen shoulder
Another common symptom of the aging person is the so-called frozen shoulder. The causes may be numerous. Unfortunately there is still no effective cure for this condition. However the chiropractor is able to make a diagnosis, establish the cause relieve the pain and improve the freedom of movement of the shoulder joint.

Headache and neck pain
Headache and neck pain are common among the elderly. Painkillers are often prescribed for these symptoms. The chiropractor can do more about these symptoms, primarily by treating the upper part of the spinal column and the neck. Dizziness too can thus be treated.

Decalcification of the vertebrae (osteoporosis)
Backache is often the result of decalcification of the spinal vertebrae. The chiropractor is able to assess the severity of the symptom, often with the aid of X-ray pictures and can tailor the treatment technique accordingly. This is directed towards functional improvement of the spinal column. The improved mobility lessens the pain considerably while generally the patient will feel much better.

Ankle-knee and wrist ache
Above it was stated that pain is often the result of the condition of the vertebrae. This can lead to back aches

or a sprained ankle, shoulder pain can be caused by a weak wrist which may also be the cause of pain in the neck. Often these pains are not associated with the real cause because the location of the cause is far removed from the pain. The chiropractor is prepared for this and identifies the cause. Thus he may decide to treat backache originating in the knee joint via the knee. Also the patient is given advice on how to exercise at home to achieve lasting results.

Pain below the shoulder blade
Many older people complain about pain below the shoulder blade. Muscle tension can cause this pain or neuralgia in the ribs or the spinal column. The symptom can also be caused by a poor function of the gallbladder or heart muscle. Rarely the pain below the shoulder blades is accompanied by breathing problems which may give rise to chest symptoms. Needless to say the right diagnosis is of vital importance. Most disturbances can be diagnosed and treated by the chiropractor.

Degenerative diseases
Degenerative diseases are diseases due to a reduced action of the vital functions. Decline is in fact inherent to aging. A common degenerative condition is osteoporosis, thinning of the bones due to diminished activity of the osteoblasts, the cell at the bone surface that produce the bone tissue. In osteoporosis the natural destruction of bone tissue is increased, resulting in pain and often skeleton deformation and sponta-

neous fractures. There are other 'degenerative symptoms' that will not be discussed here. X-ray pictures facilitate tracing the origin of the symptoms, so the chiropractor tailor the treatment schema to the needs of the patient.

Facial neuralgia
As you are well aware of the chiropractor focuses on the treatment of the central nervous system. Damage to the jaw (maxillary joint) can result in facial neuralgia (pains). Different causes may be involved. Even a poor fitting set of dentures may be the culprit. Other, less obvious, causes may lead to facial neuralgia. If required the chiropractor will refer the patient to the dentist.

And cancer…?
It is advisable to have regular check-ups by a chiropractor. When the cause of possible pain is not directly found X-rays of the skeleton will be taken. Sometimes cancer at an early stage will be detected. This greatly increases the chances of recovery, although we do not claim that that the chiropractor is able to treat cancer. We mention cancer in this chapter on chiropractic and the elderly because cancer is prevalent in older people.

When de chiropractor detects cancer he will refer the patient to the family doctor who in his turn will refer the patient to a specialist. The chiropractor can be of assistance in reducing the pain caused by cancer.

Severe back symptoms
Of course the chiropractor is the right therapist to treat back symptoms. The treatment involves manipulation in the way described above. In rare instances an operation is required. The chiropractor will refer the patient to the surgeon. It happens more and more that he surgeon first gets in touch with the chiropractor to discuss the nature and severity of the symptom. Naturally the chiropractor will always try to prevent surgery.

Posture and exercise
Growing older often involves that people become less active. People no longer go to work, walk and cycle less, so all in all people get insufficient physical exercise in old age. Thus we sit too often in uncomfortable chairs, lie on poor beds and assume the wrong posture during daily chores. The latter also holds for younger people but since the activities of older people are more limited, so are their movements. We know that back and joints symptoms are often related to poor work end living conditions. Thus the question is: *'How do we maintain a good physical condition as long as possible?'*

Sadly it turns out that everybody aspires to attain this but that few are willing to actually do something about it. The result is pain and painkillers, the latter causing further symptoms.

Summary common symptoms

- Ankle-knee-wrist pain
- Arthritis hip joint
- Backache
- Breathing problems
- Decalcification of vertebrae
- Degenerative disorders
- Dizziness
- Facial neuralgia
- Frozen shoulder
- Gallbladder, poor function
- Headache
- Heart muscle, poor function
- Joint inflammation
- Muscle strain
- Neck symptoms
- Neuralgia
- Pain
- Rheumatic disorders
- Shoulder blade-pain below
- Stiff joints

The chiropractor offers a path to better health and combats pain without drugs. Thus the aging individual is presented with an excellent alternative with regard to the symptoms mentioned above. The chiropractor will also offer the patient sound advice about proper posture and the right kind of exercise.

He can offer advice about healthy food, a better bed, a proper chair and a better way of working, both at home and outside. Because of this the aging person will stay healthy and active well into old age.

13. Stress and chiropractic

> *'We are accustomed to believe that*
> *environmental pollution affects*
> *our physical and mental health'*

Most of us are confronted with various forms of environmental pollution. Although we resist it life in a poor environment is regarded as normal and inevitable. Of course a number of environmental factors are impossible or hard to control and we have become accustomed to the fact that many of these factors affect our health. We are thus used to the idea that the poor environment simply affects our physical and mental health negatively.

A first step towards better health is that we become aware of the risks affect our existence in this context. Only then we'll be able to control and reverse these bad influences.

Structural elements in our environment

First we have to deal in our daily life with the so-called *structural* elements in our environment. Tables, chairs, beds can be causes of physical strain. These elements influence our posture. We know that a poor posture can be the cause of various symptoms, which are usually not associated with these objects. Fortunately by applying certain changes we can positively influence the quality of our daily environment. A better bed can for example have a positive effect on posture during sleep while symptoms like insomnia, restlessness and fatigue at rising greatly improve with a healthy matrass.

Daily we are exposed to still other elements affecting our health. We inhale cigarette smoke and exhaust fumes, and we consume food with chemical additives of all kinds. Obviously these elements affect our physical health negatively.

Since the effect extends over a long period and, so, does not cause immediate problems, it constitutes an insidious danger rather than a clear and present danger.

> *'People who lead a harmonious and happy life, without worry or stress, are less prone to health problems than those who lead a trouble existence'*

Every day we are faced with psychological problems: emotional problems at work or at home, little or no relaxation. Sometimes there are money troubles, guilt feelings after a broken affair, sorrow, hope or longing. Hardly a day goes by when we do not have to deal with emotions. Naturally these emotions affect our mental health which is closely linked to our physical health. A familiar example is stomach ulcer resulting from mental strain which may of course give rise to many other symptoms. People who lead a harmonious and happy life, without worry or stress, are less prone to health problems than those who lead a troubled existence.

The nervous system
There are primitive life forms in which a single cell controls all vital functions, such as the amoeba. At the other extreme is the human body, one of the most complex forms of life. Organisms have evolved, cells have specialized (*differentiated*) and constitute special organs with different functions like the brain, heart, lungs, etc. This gave rise to the need for a single system controlling and co-ordinating all bodily functions: the nervous system.

The nervous system, consisting of the brain and the spinal cord, is a complex and vulnerable system. It is protected against outside influences by a number of bones: the skull and spinal column. A very important task if we realize that the nervous system responds to outside stimuli, transmitting these stimuli to our brain. This process is the basis for our actions and thought. The body reacts to these stimuli every second of our existence.

The environment
Because life around us, the environment, is changing all the time the senses are 'bombarded' by stimuli. The senses constantly receive new stimuli, forcing us to respond. In order to prevent being overtaxed the nervous system has learnt to adept to these constant changes.

A healthy person is expected to weather through the daily challenges, disappointments and other troubles. But even the person liable to suffer from stress is able to withstand these stimuli. But sometimes things go wrong.

The symptoms
Gradually the pressure may become too great and the number of stimuli greater than our nervous system can handle. Sometimes we experience this consciously, sometimes subconsciously. In any case we receive warning signals from the nervous system that tell us that we are at risk of being overburdened. The straw that broke the camel's back. Since we are used to pressures and stress, emotions and sorrow, we are inclined to ignore these warnings. The nervous system protests against this and changes its tack.

Symptoms of stress

* Insomnia
* Restlessness
* Fatigue
* Guilt feelings
* Grief, hope, longing
* Disappointment
* Headache
* Nervousness
* Apathy
* Depression
* Disinterestedness
* Feelings of helplessness
* Lack of libido
* Panic attacks
* Lack of appetite
* Decreased activity
* Various symptoms

At first only seemingly innocuous symptoms arise like feelings of unease, feeling queer, overtiredness, feelings of discomfort or dissatisfaction. But we are told that these feelings are normal. They are part of our hectic existence of our demanding jobs, of the poor environment, etc. Usually we continue down this path or take a holiday 'just to charge our batteries'.

In short, we place these feelings under the heading 'stress' and try to make the best of it. But the nervous system doesn't put up with it and sends more and more warning signals. Then new symptoms arise like headache, nervousness, apathy, depression, disinterestedness, feelings of helplessness or panic, lack of appetite, decreased activity. There comes a time that we no longer no how to react to our feelings and symptoms.

Unfortunately stress symptoms are not properly recognized by our environment. There is little support for the patient suffering from stress. Family and colleagues are at a loss or believe it is just all part of the job ,there's no escape from it. Only when the syndrome (pattern of symptoms) call out for action the *symptoms* are treated. The pharmaceutical industry has an answer for any symptom. The patient is given *anti-stress drugs* like painkillers, tranquilizers. Through this the symptoms are suppressed but the cause of the problem is not tackled and besides, the patient is now *feeling fine*. Tranquilizers make you calm (tranquil), the negative feelings disappear and one is made to believe everything is fine again. While the real cause has not disappeared! This is just being temporarily suppressed. The result is that the patient eventually can't do without these suppressing drugs and becomes addicted to them.

A chiropractic idea

Let us represent a healthy and harmonious person by an equilateral triangle. There is a chemical side, a mental side and a structural side. As long as the right balance is maintained everything is fine. When one side is off balance then the two others too will get out of balance. Suppose we are under great mental strain, for example by job-related events. Then the *mental side* is off balance.

A harmonious person stands in the middle of:
1. Chemical side
2. Mental side
3. Structural side

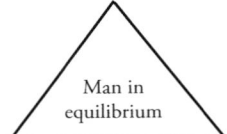
Man in equilibrium

As a result of this the *chemical side* too becomes unbalanced. This may result in increased susceptibility for colds, flu, etc. The structural side too may be thrown off balance. Backache for example may occur. Symptoms may arise that hardly or not at all seem related to the actual cause of stress: the unpleasant job-related circumstances.

In chiropractic the individual health is viewed from the so-called holistic viewpoint. That means that our health is 'designed' in perfect balance just like the well-balanced triangle. Physical energy flows freely throughout the body and controls the proper functioning of organs and tissues. Originally this balance is perfect. When this balance is disturbed then parts of the energy flow may become blocked, resulting in the afore-mentioned symptoms or other symptoms. Disease may now develop. In other words: when something is wrong with our mental condition the body can never stay healthy. When the body becomes ill chances are that the mental state deteriorates further: thus a vicious circle develops.

> *'Symptoms may arise that are hardly or not at all related to the actual cause of stress'*

The chiropractor focuses on the overall picture. For him/her all factors carry the same weight. This means in fact that to begin with an attempt is made to find the root cause and only then an effective treatment is initiated. The chiropractor may be expected to identify the nature of the complaint: is the cause of the symptom *structural*, *mental* or *chemical*? Simply to treat the symptom would just be treatment of symptoms. This should definitely be avoided. Then the symptoms would only temporarily disappear, something that is not much help to the patient.

The chiropractor also offers advice to the patient. *Don't be too sure nothing can be done about the situation at work or in the home.* The solution is often so close at hand that one easily overlooks it. Perhaps unnecessarily we repeat that the chiropractor's treatment does not involve drugs. So addiction to synthetic drugs is excluded from the very start.

What can the chiropractor do?
Above it was shown that stress may give rise to *mechanical* symptoms. Especially the spinal column can be affected. The chiropractor is able to establish a precise diagnosis and treat *mechanical* and *structural* symptoms related to joints, spinal column and the

effects on the nervous system. A specially designed treatment scheme is aimed at removing the actual cause i.e. the cause of the energy blockade, so the energy can once more circulate freely throughout the body. Also, symptoms apparently not associated with the actual cause may disappear. The patient is expected to follow the chiropractor's advice at home to make sure the symptoms do not recur.

Structural symptoms such as low backache, shoulder pain or sciatica are usually treated by drugs like painkillers in conventional medicine. Sometimes surgery is recommended. But increasingly doctors refer the patient to the chiropractor, a development that is bound to continue. Another positive point is that doctors increasingly focus on the cause of a symptom and centre their attention on differentiate between structural, chemical and mental symptoms. The emphasis is on diagnostics, the starting point for treatment and recovery.

14. Most common pains and chiropractic

*'Sometimes patients are resigned to
having to live with backache,
but it remains quite a challenge'*

The chiropractor is the therapist per excellence for neck, shoulder and back symptoms and related symptoms. In this chapter we'll discuss the most common pain symptoms. Statistics show that at least one-third of the population occasionally or permanently suffers from backache or headache. Many people suffer from this condition for years, even decades. Sometimes people are resigned to having to live with backache, but it remains quite a challenge. It may affect our daily functioning. Often they turn from one therapist to another, usually to no avail.

Backache is not a disease
Let us just consider what backache may involve. In any case pain in the back is not an illness per se. Backache is a sign that there is a disturbance in the body. After examination it turns out that in most cases there is a mechanical disturbance. This disturbance can be due to changes of the normal mobility of the joints. The spinal column doesn't function optimally, the nervous system is irritated and backache develops. One is often inclined to call it 'strained muscles', a cold, rheumatism, muscle in-

flammation, arthritis, hernia, sciatica and even kidney problems.

In any case backache is usually accompanied by decreased mobility, whereby each movement produces more pain. With disturbances within the spinal column pain can be felt elsewhere in the body which is often not associated with the disturbance in the spinal column. Pain may occur in the arms or legs, neck, shoulders, head, shoulder blades, even in the breast.

This book has discussed the cause of backache, i.e. disturbances inside the spinal column, for example, always moving wrongly in the exercise of one's activities. This does not necessarily imply heavy physical labour, but also sitting on a poor office chair can be a cause. The disturbance can occur as a result of a fall, accident, thrust, or even prolonged coughing. A sudden movement can be the cause but also sleeping on a poor matrass. Adopting a wrong posture may also be a causal connection.

It turns out that the disturbance may develop in the course of years or that the disturbance may occur suddenly (as a result of an accident or fall for example). The acute disturbance directly identifies its origin. In this situation the disturbance has been caused by a wrong movement during work or sport. When the pain in the back continues the cause is easily identified and treatment can start immediately. Disturbances that develop slowly over time are the ones that are often ignored. The severity of the symptom may depend on a number of factors. The general condition may play a role, the patient's age, build, muscle tone, profession and working conditions. In most cases the patient experiences pain at the lower end of the back, not so strange when one realizes that the lumbar vertebrae bear the greatest weight of the body. Tension at the lower end of the back can affect the normal functioning of the joints. This is at the expense of the mobility of the joints and the natural flexibility can change because of this. Then extra strain is put on joints, muscles and intervertebral discs, resulting in more pain.

> *'The general condition may play a role, the patient's age, build, muscle tone, profession and working conditions'*

What can be done to prevent backache (due to disturbances in the spinal column) and other symptoms will be discussed in chapter 20, *How to prevent symptoms yourself.* Apart for sparing your back it is advisable to be aware of any possible disturbances within the spinal column. It should be realized that damage of the intervertebral discs is relatively common in people between 30 and 50 years of age. At these ages the person has quite a bit of work experience behind him/her. Wrong actions /movements during work may have resulted in the gradual development of back symptoms.

Sciatica

A common symptom seen by the chiropractor is sciatica. A symptom commonly caused by defects, damage, or irritation at the location where the biggest nerve (sciatic nerve) leaves the spinal cord. This nerve runs from the lumbar region all the way to the toes.

The pain may be unilateral or bilateral and may be felt at any stretch along the sciatic nerve; along the hips, or along the thighs, calves, feet and toes. Other symptoms too may suggest sciatica, like numbness, impaired blood circulation, tingling in the feet and even partial paralysis.

Just like similar back symptoms sciatica may result from a fall, lifting a heavy object the wrong way, straining or a wrongly assumed posture. In short, when circumstances occur resulting in a gradual or sudden strain in the lumbar region sciatica can develop. Age as well as strenuous work conditions and a deformed spinal column may be contributing factors. Even pregnancy may be a cause of sciatica.

Other symptoms

As mentioned there are many symptoms that at first sight are unrelated to the spine. Still these symptoms may actually be regarded as *related symptoms.* Everyone has occasionally suffered from neck pain or neck stiffness. We dismiss these symptoms as 'having slept in the wrong position' or tiredness. We keep quiet for a little while and the pain disappears. Possibly the symptom may well be of an innocuous nature. But always be aware that the neck is the most vulnerable part of the spinal column. Most people are not sufficiently aware of this. These seemingly innocuous symptoms may well result in a serious symptom if we pay too little attention to it. If we are aware of the possible risks we're on the right track. It is all a matter of recognizing the symptoms and their potential for lasting damage. The nature of these signals is hard to describe because they differ among people. The human body is a complex whole without a 'user's manual'. Tips do exist that can be seen as a pointer to a possibly serious symptom. Intense pain in the neck, shoulders or arms that persists or returns after a short or longer period. Apart from the most vulnerable part the neck is also the most sensitive part of the spinal column. The neck responds immediately to stress, exertion, strain, accidents and falls.

Pain lasting more than 24 hours should be seen as a grave warning. A visit to the chiropractor would be no luxury, even if the symptom turns out to be harmless.

Neck, shoulder and arm pains
Neck pain usually starts with a mild pain that can extend to the shoulders and/or arms. Also an intense pain can occur radiating to the shoulders and arms. This can be a symptom of the conditions mentioned below: nerve inflammation (neuritis), bursitis (inflammation of the bursa), nerve pains (neuralgia), rheumatism, the so-called *frozen shoulder* or fibrositis (inflammation of connective tissue).

Often the causes of the pain are less serious: strain of the neck muscles, inevitable effects of getting older or a poor blood circulation. There may also be pain, stiffness or diminished mobility without discernible cause. Further, there are symptoms unrelated to the condition of the neck as such, but which do affect the neck. We may mention irritated nerves in the neck or surroundings, face ears, head. The neck may even be related to stiffness and numbness in the fingers, tingling fingers, loss of balance, a certain tension in the eyes or migraine.

Neck symptoms can be caused in the same way as back symptoms, they can develop slowly or suddenly because of a wrong posture or poor working conditions, a fall or a thrust, an accident or a wrong move during sport. Whichever factor causes neck symptoms, the result can be that the seven neck vertebrae no longer function properly and no longer perform their duties. Nerves can even be completely blocked or become irritated. In both cases this results in pain, irritation and /or stiffness. If treatment is not initiated there will be a risk of serious damage. It can be the start of bone and joint inflammation.

Headache
Apart from backache headache is a common symptom at all ages. No less than fifteen percent of all patients seeking help from a chiropractor suffers from headache. Sometimes occasionally, with longer short intervals, sometimes constantly. There are many 'kinds' of headache with as many causes. Fortunately most headaches are innocuous and can be treated by an aspirin. The occasional use of aspirin can do little harm. The less innocuous kinds of headache may point to a disturbance in the body. Here too, kinds of pain that apparently are not related to the actual cause. Once again pain that is too often accepted as 'normal', which we simply have to endure. Still it is of great importance to find the cause. Most headaches can definitely be effectively treated.

Just as with backache headache may be caused by different factors. The nature of headache can vary widely. Sometimes the headache radiates towards the temples or eyes. Sometimes the pain is felt all over the head, or part of the head. The pain can be mild or intense, of short duration or protracted. Also the pain can be just occasional or frequent.

Headache can result from stress and/or nervousness, but also from taut muscles, overtiredness, overexertion, anxiety or other stress symptoms. Headache caused by stress in the most common pain. This type of headache is commonly the result of the contraction of the neck muscles, especially at the base of the skull. As a reaction to this contraction pain in the head can be felt, but also in the neck or back. Symptoms of this type of headache are usually pain just behind the forehead, pain at both temples, pain above or behind the eyes and pressure on the temples. Being on edge or a sense of discomfort can be a sign that a headache is coming on. In some patients all these symptoms occur, in others just a few.

The deeper cause
The head is supported by two short bundles of muscles attached to the lower part of the scull. Every distortion or block of these muscles or other muscles at the top of the neck can mean that the muscles are in a constant state of contraction. This affects the natural balance of the head. Normally these muscles at the top of the neck enable greater movement than other

vertebral connections. Because of this these vertebrae are vulnerable and easily damaged. So the surrounding muscles can easily contract (spasm), which can result in headache. There may be other causes. A fall can lead to problems involving muscle groups. This also applies to blows or thrusts, the so-called whip-lash, a poor posture or emotional stress. Wrong moves van also cause pain in the head or neck. The neck muscles are not only of importance for balancing the head, they are also required cushioning daily movements like thrusts and thus prevent problems lower in the spinal column.

Migraine
Migraine, too, sometimes appears to the patient like an *intangible* symptom about little can be done. Justifiably it is said that migraine has so many causes that tackling it is futile from the start. There may be a *throbbing pain* on one side of the head or pain due to a glaring light. Migraine is often accompanied by queasiness. Migraine can be preceded by visual disturbances like spots or/and flashes of light.

Sometimes migraine is found in several members of the family, which suggests a hereditary factor. Finally, migraine often occurs at waking up or after eating certain kinds of food (cheese, chocolate) or drinking wine.

What is migraine?
Visual disturbances result from the contraction of blood vessels running towards the head. In response

these blood vessels are causing pain. Sometimes the cause is a disturbance in the spinal column. The nervous system responsible for the blood vessels is then damaged. The system is disordered and migraine is one of its symptoms.

When the cause is in the spinal column the chiropractor can correct the disturbance. He/she focuses on that part of the spinal column where the disturbance is located. Usually the pain disappears after a series of treatments or eases considerably. In any case an in-depth diagnosis is made exploring all possible causes.

The medical history is also considered and possibly the chiropractor will make use of X-ray pictures of the spinal column and the surrounding muscle groups. Where the nervous system is damaged and where the nerves no longer exert full control over the blood vessels adjustments are carried out. The number of treatments depends on the nature and severity of the symptom. If migraine results from the use of certain kinds of food or drinks then the chiropractor will confine himself to giving advice about which foods and drinks to avoid. If it turns out that the cause cannot be treated by the chiropractor then the patient will be referred to another therapist, family doctor or specialist.

Most common symptoms

* Pain in the back
* Sciatica
* Pain in the neck
* Pain in shoulders or arms
* Headache
* Migraine

15. Training of the chiropractor

'In the UK it is illegal to call oneself a Chiropractor. It is a legal requirement to be registered with the General Chiropractic Council'

This chapter express the schooling of the chiropractor. It should be of interest to the patient to learn what the training of the reliable chiropractor entails.

Like any university study the study of chiropractic is an arduous one. High demands are made on preparatory training. In the UK there are three chiropractic colleges recognised by the General Chiropractic Council.

When the student meets the condition of the preparatory training, he/she can be accepted at the *Anglo-European College of Chiropractic* (AECC) in Bournemouth. Furthermore, the student may be accepted at the *McTimoney College of Chiropractic*. The MCC offers an Undergraduate Masters Degree in human chiropractic and two post-graduate masters programmes in animal manipulation as well as a master programme in paediatric chiropractic. Also the Welsh Institute of Chiropractic (WIOC - University of Glamorgan) offers a M.Chiro programme ('Health Sciences including Nursing and Chiropractic').

- In the UK it is illegal to call oneself a Chiropractor.
- It is a legal requirement to be registered with the

General Chiropractic Council (GCC).
- In order to retain registration a minimum of 30 hours p.a. continuing professional development is required.
- The UK-degrees: Master of Chiropractic (MC) or Master in Chiropractic (M.Chiro).
- Chiropractic is governed internationally by the Councils on Chiropractic Education International (CCEI).
- The CCEI is recognized by the World Federation of Chiropractic and the World Health Organization.

Theoretical subjects combined with practical subjects
During the first three years of the full-time education of four years of study, theoretical subjects are combined with a few practical subjects. Towards the final year the student gains practical experience. Students are spending 4200 'student-teacher' contact hours (classroom, clinical experience and laboratory), including a minimum of 1000 supervised clinical training hours.

Next to the subjects chosen
After this the subjects chosen will be explained but courses are also given on chiropractic philosophy, the chiropractic clinic, measuring instruments, various techniques, science of law, economics, ethics. Anatomy and neurology are two important main subjects.

Study package
The following long list of subjects is not complete and can be adapted to needs. The list does make clear that the level of the chiropractic studies is very high.

1 Anatomy
Anatomy for the sake of knowledge of the exterior and interior of man.

2 Theory of the inorganic
Theory of the non-organic (for example cardiac murmur not caused by organ abnormalities).

3 Bacteriology
Science of bacteria, examination for the presence of bacteria.

4 Biochemistry
The science that studies the application of chemistry to biology.

5 Diagnostics
Knowledge of diagnosis, the art of making a diagnosis.

6 Dietetics.
Nutrition, for example prescribing food which differs for medical reasons from the usual food.

7 Dissection
Study of the (dead) human body, dissecting tissues.

8 First Aid
First aid in the case of accidents (acting fast and efficiently in an emergency).

9 Physiotherapy
Medical treatment of orthopaedic, neurological, rheumatic-psychogenic abnormalities of the (normal) posture and function.

- Orthopaedic: study of the prevention and treatment of pathological abnormalities of the locomotor apparatus.
- Neurological: study of somatic disorders of the nervous system and their treatment.
- Psychogenic: finding the cause within the soul.

10 Hygiene
Also denoted by: general / individual / public hygiene. It is the study of health, food, bathing, clothing, night rest, movement.

11 Gynaecology
Science of the disorders of the female sex organs.

12 Histology
Histopathology is the study of pathological changes in organic tissues.

13 Laboratory
Workplace for empirical –scientific or technical studies and experiments.

14 Myology
Study of muscles

15 Neurophysiology
Study of the vital functions relating to the nervous system.

16 Neurology
Science/study of the somatic (physical) disorders of the nervous system and their treatment.

17 Science of the organic
The study of organs.

18 Orthopaedics
Subdivision of surgery concerned with the prevention and treatment of pathological form and function abnormalities of the active and passive locomotor system.

19 Osteology
Study of bones.

20 Pathology
Study of diseases.

21 Psychiatry
The study of mental diseases

22 Psychology
The science concerned with the study of consciousness and related phenomena.

23 Radiology
The study of radioactivity in medicine and of the application of radiation energy in diagnostics and therapy.

24 Roentgenology
Science of the application of roentgen rays for diagnostics and therapy.

25 Chemistry
Study of the properties and composition of substances and their changes.

26 Spinography
Study of the spinal column and analysing X-rays for chiropractic purposes.

27 Symptomatology
Study of symptoms, the totality of signs of a given disease.

28 Toxicology
Study of toxins.

29 Obstetrics
Study of childbirth and its proper management.

30 Vitaminology
Study of vitamins, trace elements, organic substances present in food in tiny amounts, essential for the proper maintenance of normal metabolism.

Summary prerequisite classes

* Analytical chemistry
* Biochemistry
* Biomechanics
* Cellular biology
* Embryology
* Exercise physiology
* General chemistry
* Genetics
* Human anatomy
* Immunology
* Kinesiology
* Microbiology
* Nuclear medicine
* Nutrition
* Organic chemistry
* Pharmacology
* Physics
* Physiology
* Statistics
* Toxicology

16. Movements within chiropractic

'The 'mixed' chiropractors constitute the modern variants. They mix other techniques with their therapy, make a clinical diagnosis whenever possible'

Just as there are different opinions about sickness and health within conventional medicine, so there are different views within chiropractic. This is not about conflicts within chiropractic and the patient should not worry about not getting proper treatment. We'll present a brief description of these trends.

Straight or mixed?
A distinction can be made between the so-called 'straight' and 'mixed' chiropractors. Straight chiropractors focus mainly on identifying and correcting the 'subluxation'. In general they do not make a real clinical diagnosis and they adhere closely to the original theories of D.D. Palmer. 'Philosophy' is of paramount importance to them and their treatment is virtually confined to manipulation techniques. This group makes little use of therapeutic exercises and myofascial treatment techniques. Myofascial therapy is aimed at the treatment of symptoms of (incorrect) posture and the locomotor apparatus.

According to the straight chiropractors virtually all diseases can be reduced to disturbances in the spinal column, a view that may have been plausible in 1895, but no longer.

Modern variant
The 'mixed' chiropractors constitute the modern variant. They mix other techniques in their therapy, make whenever possible a clinical diagnosis and do not limit themselves exclusively to correcting subluxations. Actually, the terms 'subluxation 'and 'innate intelligence' (life force) derived from Palmer 's original theories are considered unscientific and incomplete by this school. Mixed chiropractors are receptive to a professional dialogue with conventional professionals and harbour the ambition to achieve a recognized position within conventional medical care. Mixed chiropractors are more nuanced in their claims about effectiveness and confine their field of activity to symptoms of the locomotor apparatus, like low-back pain, neck and headache symptoms, sport injuries, etc. No claims are made about the effectiveness of treatment in the case of organic conditions and other diseases.

'Both in the sphere of treatment, diagnosis, philosophy, scientific underpinning and explanation differences between these schools clearly exist'

The group of mixed chiropractors is predominant. According to this school, mixed chiropractic is a necessary professional development to ensure being taken seriously as a professional group in the future.

Specialisations
Within chiropractic specialization are possible in the fields functional neurology, paediatrics, sport, orthopaedics and radiology. This concerns schooling aimed at providing supplementary knowledge and competence in specific fields.

In his original theories Palmer spoke of *crooked vertebrae* causing 'nerves to become wedged'. As a result the flow of *innate intelligence* (life force) was impeded with all kind of consequences for the functioning of organs and health. Since there are MRI scanners we know that a vertebra is not easily displaced and that under normal circumstances nerves do not get jammed. This explanation is obsolete and is no longer accepted by modern chiropractors. The correct explanation of a functional spinal lesion is related to local neurophysiological effects, and its neurological consequences. The *displaced vertebra* and the 'manually pushing back or adjusting by the chiropractor ' is no longer valid today. A manipulation only affects the mobility of the joint and the associated neurophysiological abnormalities, but the position of the vertebra remains unchanged.

> *'In the case of 'normal' back symptoms*
> *the cause of the pain is rarely*
> *found in X-ray pictures'*

X-ray pictures have played a big part in the early years of chiropractic. Today most chiropractors make less use of X-ray, because the X-ray picture is not suitable for detecting a functional abnormality in the spinal column. After all, a functional disturbance is a mobility problem, and so cannot be seen in a stationary picture in the form of a X-ray picture or MRI. In the case of 'normal' back symptoms the cause of pain is rarely found in X-ray pictures. Chiropractors still use X-ray usually, especially in order to exclude contra-indications for treatment or pathology.

17. Summary: which symptoms?

*'Often chiropractic yields results where
other methods bring no relief'*

Many health problems can be alleviated or resolved by a chiropractic treatment. Experience shows that this holds both for acute problems and chronic conditions. Chiropractic focuses on the treatment of symptoms, on 'maintenance' of treated symptoms and on prevention.

This chapter presents the most common symptoms for which the chiropractor is consulted.

The most common symptoms the chiropractor treats concern the back, shoulders and neck. Headache, migraine, facial pain, and tingling and numbness in arms and legs are also common. Pain and stiffness, e.g. due to arthritis, can diminish greatly by chiropractic treatment. Women with low-back pain or menstrual pain can benefit from chiropractic assistance. Also 'whiny babies' and symptoms like bed-wetting in children can often be treated successfully.

Also symptoms outside the spinal column can be treated: aching or stiff muscles and joint pains, for example in the elbows (tennis arm), knees, ankles and feet. Sometimes in the case of arthritis pain relief and functional improvement of the joints can be achieved.

Because the organs and tissues require an undisturbed nervous supply to function properly it is not hard to understand that many functional disturbances respond favourably to chiropractic. This also holds for 'vague' symptoms like dizziness, fatigue and listlessness: the cause may be located in the spinal column.

Low-back symptoms

Low-back pain is very common. Problems in the lower back may manifest themselves in different ways. Many people complain about a nagging pain or a stiff back, but the pain can also be felt as nerve pain, for example radiating to the legs.

Anatomy of the back
The lower back consists of five lumbar vertebrae. Between each of these is an intervertebral disc. The intervertebral disc functions as a shock absorber. At the back the vertebrae are mutually connected by two joints, one on the left and one on the right. Several muscles run along the spinal column, which enable us for example to sit and walk upright and move about.

The pelvis constitutes the base on which the spinal column rests and carries the body weight. The pelvis consists of a central triangular part (the sacrum) which forms a joint on both sides with the two hipbones. These joints are held together by strong ligaments.

Symptoms
The symptoms that arise in the lower back are dependent on the local structure. The muscles, the joints, and the intervertebral discs at the level of the lumbar vertebrae can cause symptoms. Despite the fact that the symptoms may appear virtually identical the causes can be different. The right diagnosis is very important and because different causes require different treatments sufficient time must be allotted for examination.

Causes of low back pain or pelvis pain can be classified as gradually coming on or acute.

Gradually arising causes are
- Little change in posture and little exercise (for example office work)
- Wrong and one-sided load (regularly lifting the wrong way)
- Natural aging of the cartilage in the neck (arthrosis, due to wear or degeneration)
- Stress, fatigue, illness, cold, moisture, etc.
- Changes in hormone levels during pregnancy

Acute causes can be
- Traffic accident
- Wrong move or twist

Upper back and shoulder symptoms

The upper back is the part of the back where the vertebrae are connected to the ribs. Pain in the back can be accompanied by stiffness and pain in other locations in the back, the neck or chest.

Symptoms
When there are problems in the upper back it can lead to various symptoms. Most people with upper back symptoms experience pain between the shoulder blades. But pain in the chest or radiating pain in the arms can also be the result of an upper back problem. Sometimes the symptoms mimic heart symptoms and this often causes anxiety. Coughing, sneezing and breathing can be painful. The chiropractor can determine if the symptoms are related to a back problem.

Causes
Backache may have several causes. Pain in the upper back usually develops gradually, as a result of an incorrect posture (sitting behind the desk the wrong way), one-sided use of the arms by always making the same movement (such as ironing) and working a lot overhead. Rarely, pain in the upper back has an acute cause, like straining oneself or a wrong move. One or more vertebrae in the wrong position (e.g. jammed) may cause strain in the upper back. Nerves become irritated and that causes pain. Even problems in organs, for example gastric complaints, may be associated with irritated nerves in the back.

Treatment
The first thing the chiropractor does is ask questions about the back complaints and the general state of health, since the backache can be related to other health problems. This is followed by a physical examination. The chiropractor makes use of various medical methods to determine where the pain arises and the

mobility of all vertebrae that may be involved. Sometimes X-ray pictures are made. The chiropractor applies pressure techniques to the spinal column. Their objective is to remove blockades and disturbances, so nerves, muscles and vertebrae can again function normally.

Apart from applying pressure techniques it is possible that the patient are prescribed exercises. Advice about posture or diet may be part of the treatment.

Prevention
Prevention gets a lot of attention in chiropractic. It is quite possible that the chiropractor advises to return regularly to check the spinal column in order to prevent the complaints from returning or getting worse. But the patient himself/herself too can contribute to structural improvement of the problems.

A good position while standing or sitting prevents back symptoms. It is also important to move in a responsible manner in order to prevent overtaxing or straining oneself. The chiropractor can offer advice. Questions like 'which sport would be best for me and with which I specially should be careful about', will be answered by the chiropractor.

Neck and shoulder complaints

Common conditions are: stiffness of the neck and shoulder muscles, whiplash, muscle pain, arthritis and neck hernia.

Symptoms
The most common neck complaints are nagging pain and stiffness. Neck pain can develop gradually as a result of strained muscles in the neck and shoulder girdle, but also suddenly, for example due to a wrong move. This is often accompanied by headache.

Other possible complaints are
- Dizziness and ringing ears
- Concentration problems
- Radiating pain to the arms
- Feeling of tiredness or weakness in shoulders and arms
- Tingling in hands or fingers

Causes
These symptoms too can develop slowly but may also have an acute cause.

Gradually arising causes can be
- Little variety in the working position, like in desk work
- Little variety in moving
- Wrong or one-sided bearing load
- Natural aging of cartilage in the neck (arthritis, referred to as wear or degeneration)
- Stress
- Frequent exposure to cold and draught

Acute causes can be
- Fall or accident (this can result in whiplash)
- Muscle spasms due to a wrong movement or twist
- Wrong position during sleep
- Infection of auditory meatus or airways

Migraine

Nearly all of us suffer from headache once in a while. There are many forms of headaches, like tension headache, migraine, facial neuralgia and headache resulting from whiplash.

Migraine is a familiar kind of headache and is often confused with other forms of headache. Migraine occurs in about 1 in 10 adults. An estimated five percent of children suffers from migraine till the 11th year. Migraine is caused by changes of the diameter of blood vessels in the head, where the mobility of the neck vertebrae and irritation of the nerves may play a part. A chiropractic treatment can offer alleviation in certain forms of migraine.

Symptoms

Migraine can occur as migraine with an aura or without. Migraine without an aura is the most common form. Someone with migraine with an aura experiences neurological signs during an attack. This form starts with flashes and spots in front of the eyes and changes into a stinging pain on one side of the head. Migraine without aura has no influence on vision, but often causes headache around one eye or on one side of the face. These migraine attacks can last a couple of hours or days. Migraine can result in nausea and vomiting. During a migraine attack one may be oversensitive to light and sound.

Causes

Much is still unclear about the cause of migraine. While it was considered to be a problem of the blood vessels until the recent past, we now know that it is a neurological disorder. The blood vessels respond to the wrong stimulation by dilating. This can result in a throbbing or piercing headache. Migraine also appears to have a hereditary cause. Certain foods, drugs, alcohol can also trigger a migraine attack. Examples are wine, chocolate or cheese. In women migraine is often associated with the menstrual cycle. No wonder the prevalence of migraine in women is three times higher than in men, possibly because of different hormone levels and their effect on the blood vessels. The chiropractor examines whether a connection exists between migraine and problems with the vertebrae, joints or nerves.

Possible causes of migraine
- Irritation of blood vessels
- Foods (wine, chocolate, cheese, coffee, nitrates, sweeteners)
- Hormone level (menstrual cycle)
- Heridity
- Contraceptive pill
- Altered sleeping pattern
- Great exertion
- Sudden change in the weather
- Bright light/noises
- Cigarette/cigar smoke
- Changes in altitude (mountains, airplane)

Treatment
The headache may be connected with other health problems. So, a thorough physical examination is essential. The chiropractor uses various medical methods to establish the cause of the pain and to assess the mobility of the joints that may be involved. A chiro-

practic treatment may be useful but the chiropractor may also advise the patient to consult the family doctor for further examination.

When the symptom can be treated then muscles and nerves can function better by the application of pressure techniques. Mobility improves, muscles relax while nervous function is normalized. As a result pain and other symptoms may decrease or disappear. The result of the treatment depends on the severity of the complaints. Besides the treatment the chiropractor may offer advice about proper position, sport, exercises and diet.

Headache

Tension headache is the most common form of headache. A chiropractic treatment can often be effective.

Symptoms
Tension headache is an oppressive pain which is often described as 'splitting headache' The pain may be bilateral or on one side. Symptoms may be present all during the day, but may also develop slowly in the course the day. Tension headache may also arise from the maxillary joint. In that case the pain is usually on one side of the head. Sometimes the headache may last for days. Tension headache is often chronic and may occur periodically without regularity.

Causes
Pain usually arises from the neck and can result from wrong moves of the vertebrae in back and neck. This

overloads muscles and irritates surrounding nerves, resulting in headache. Tension headache is also related to stress and fatigue.

Treatment
Tension headache too can be connected with other health problems. If this is the case a thorough physical examination follows. The chiropractor makes use of various medical methods to establish the source of the pain and assesses the mobility of joints that might be involved.

Dependent on the complaint the chiropractor can start with the treatment. Thanks to pressure techniques the mobility improves and the muscles relax, resulting in the pain and other complaints lessening or disappearing. The result of the treatment obviously depends on the nature and severity of the symptoms.

The chiropractor can also offer advice about proper position (posture), sport, exercises and diet. Both for prevention as well as healing exercise is highly recommended. Making the wrong moves may actually make the symptoms worse. Developing strong back and neck muscles is important. This spares the spinal column and decreases the risk of the complaint returning.

Arthritis - wear

Arthritis is a joint condition that can arise as a result of the aging process. It is related to the stiffening of cartilage and occurs mostly in the back (the intervertebral discs), the knee and the hip. Of course the aging process cannot be turned back but the chiropractor can lessen pain and stiffness and slow down the aging process.

Symptoms
Restricted mobility (stiffness) is the most common symptom in arthritis. Often pain is felt around the joint. When arthritis affects the spinal column the pain can radiate to arms, legs, head or chest and is sometimes accompanied by tingling. A characteristic feature of arthritis is that the pin is worst in the morning after rising or after sitting for a long time. With movement the pain usually decreases. Only when arthritis is in an advanced stage the pain persists.

Causes
With aging the flexibility of the cartilage decreases because it becomes drier and stiffer. It happens to anyone but most people are not bothered by it. There are circumstances which accelerate the wear and increase the risk of pain. For example, too little exercise, heavy physical work, a wrong posture or old injuries. As a result of stiffness and pain the patient moves less smoothly, initiating a vicious circle. Surrounding nerves and tissues (muscles, ligaments, and joint ligaments) may also become irritated. When other joints take over the function of the stiff joint they may become overburdened and cause trouble, including pain.

Treatment
After establishing the diagnosis the chiropractor draws up a treatment program. The core of the treatment is the application of pressure techniques. By applying pressure

to certain locations the joint may be corrected. More fluid enters the joint which makes moving easier. Moreover, everything around the joint (nerves, muscles, joint ligaments) is readjusted, reducing the pain. Muscles can again relax and the patient moves a lot easier. Even severe forms of arthritis can thus be considerably relieved.

The patient, too, can contribute to keeping his joints flexible. The chiropractor will prescribe exercises to help the patient move more carefully (during work or sports). Also attention will be given to better position (posture) and diet. The patient's own commitment contributes to no small extent to the success of the treatment.

Prevention
Getting enough exercise is the best remedy against arthritis, *both* as prevention and as cure. Moving wrong can make the symptoms worse. Calm, gradual movements like walking, cycling and swimming are recommended. Sudden violent movements are best avoided.

Hernia

A hernia (*hernia nucleus pulposus*) is a bulge of an intervertebral disk and causes much pain in the back and often in both legs.

Anatomy of the intervertebral disk
Between two vertebrae lies the shock absorbing intervertebral disk, which provides elasticity and increases mobility. The intervertebral disk may be compared to an onion. Centrally located is a kind of gel

surrounded by layers. A bulge is formed when the soft inner part (*'gel'*) exerts a force on the outer layers.

The bulge presses on nerves and causes pain and other complaints. Hernia arises when the intervertebral disk loses its flexibility. This disk, which functions as *shock absorber* in the spinal column then is no longer able to effectively cushion certain movements. This results in cracks appearing in the outside of the disk as a result of which the soft inside is no longer well protected. When part of the soft gel like substance in the intervertebral disk bulges out we call it *'hernia nucleus pulposus'*. The pressure on the nerve can lead to a diminished function of the nerve.

There are no sensory nerves in the intervertebral disk. So, the hernia itself doesn't hurt. The pain is caused because the bulge presses against nervous tissue. The symptoms of hernia may differ, dependent on the nerve that is irritated. Hernia's in the lower back especially produce radiation to the legs, like tingling and numbness and can even cause paresis or creeping paralysis.

Differences between CT and MRI scan
The CT scan shows images of
* bones (often in the case of fractures)
* brain
* lungs
* abdominal organs
* arteries and veins

The MRI scan shows images of
* brain (function), spinal cord and nerves
* muscles
* ligaments and joint capsules
* heart (function)
* abdominal organs

Symptoms
Hernia causes back pain which can radiate to one or both legs. Tingling in leg or foot can also point to hernia. When the symptoms get worse the leg muscles may lose strength or become numb. In the case of a large hernia a '*cauda equina syndrome*' can arise, a condition which may cause the loss of a great number of functions, like sense of touch in the legs and control over bladder and bowel function. In that case the patient should be referred to a neurologist.

Causes
A hernia is a common condition of the lower back which produces symptoms in only fifty percent of all cases. As one grows older the intervertebral disk becomes less elastic, often resulting in weak spots in the intervertebral disks. Hernia occurs slightly more often in men than in women. Usually the cracks develop gradually as a result of incorrect position. Little variation in position (sedentary job, etc.) increases the risk of developing a hernia. The same holds for work requiring repetitive movements, like lifting, stooping a lot, and turning. Sometimes a hernia arises instantaneously as a result of an accident.

Treatment
In the case of a (possible) hernia the chiropractor will do some neurological tests. Nerves feed our muscles and skin. Each nerve has its own destination. In the case of a hernia a targeted search can be made to detect abnormalities in muscle function and/or other abnormalities. The chiropractor can conclude from the described pain radiation which nerve is affected.

The chiropractor may advise to undergo further diagnostic examination in consultation with the family doctor and neurologist. A hernia cannot be seen on an ordinary X-ray picture. Thinned intervertebral disks can be seen but that doesn't mean there is actually a hernia (bulge) present. Hernia's are clearly seen on CT or MRI scans, while the pressure of the hernia on the nerve can also be observed. If a X-ray picture, CT or MRI is available that can be useful for the chiropractor to assess the prognosis and attune the treatment accordingly.

Most hernia complaints can be effectively treated by a chiropractor without the need of an operation. By using various pressure techniques the chiropractor can to a large extent restore the spinal column's mobility, of course dependent on the nature of the symptoms. The aim is to enlarge the intervertebral disk space in order to lower the pressure of the bulge on the nerve. This can be achieved by certain *stretch or traction* techniques, exercise techniques for or muscle relaxation techniques.

In the case of a serious hernia the chiropractor may refer the patient to the family doctor or neurologist. Then, an operation may be required. However, after the operation the pain at the spot of the hernia has gone but other locations in the back or hip can still be aching. In these cases the chiropractic treatment can bring relief.

Beside the treatment with pressure techniques the chiropractor can offer advice about the right position, ergonomy, sport, exercise and diet. Even if the treatment has been effective, the back remains the weak spot that deserves attention. Developing strong abdominal, buttock and back muscles is of the greatest importance.

Whiplash
Whiplash is a quick, movement due to an accident or fall. The move can cause damage to vertebrae and tissues (muscles, nerves) in the neck. This can result in whiplash trauma: pain, stiffness and other complaints that may sometimes show only months after the accident. The chiropractor has treatment methods at his disposal to correct or alleviate whiplash symptoms.

Symptoms
The most common whiplash symptom is a painful, often stiff, neck. Many whiplash patients also suffer from headache, low back pain, and radiating pain to arms and face. But there are many other symptoms that may be part of the whiplash syndrome like loss of strength in the arms, dizziness, disturbances of equilibrium, nausea, ringing in the ears, poor vision, spots in the eyes and sleep- and concentration problems. Not only the nature, but also the severity of the symptoms varies widely. Half of the patients recover within a month, but sometimes the consequences are so serious that it leads to disability.

Causes
Whiplash is a common term that is often related to car accidents. In the past with train accidents, even small ones, people could suffer from the same pattern

of symptoms as in the case of whiplash. This was referred to as '*railway spine*'. For a long this went unrecognized and these '*railway spine victims*' received no compensation after the accident.

The term whiplash refers to a quick, forced movement of the head leading to these symptoms. So, whiplash not only occurs in traffic accidents but may result from a fall from the stairs or a skiing accident.

Since may forces are involved in a rear-end collision certain parts of the body accelerate differently. That's the reason why a whiplash accident can be so traumatic. First the torso or the lower part with the shoulders move forwards and nanoseconds later the head. As a result of this violent movement joint capsules, muscles, ligaments and nerves can be stretched causing pain and other symptoms.

Treatment
It should be established to what extent the accident may have caused the whiplash reaction. During the physical examination the chiropractor especially looks at the mobility of the joints. If whiplash is present he will assess its severity and whether it matches the severity of the symptoms. If a X-ray picture, CT or MRI is available this will be useful to make a prognosis and tune the treatment accordingly. The chiropractor can also advise to undergo further tests in consultation with the family doctor or specialist.

By carefully moving the vertebrae with the aid of pressure techniques muscles and nerves may again function normally. With the pressure techniques the mobility improves, the muscles relax, and the surrounding nerves regain their normal function. Usually pain and other complaints diminish or disappear.

Here too the chiropractor can give advice about position, ergonomics, sport, exercises and food. Moving incorrectly can make the symptoms worse. Developing strong neck muscles is very important. This spares the spinal column and lowers the risk of the symptoms returning.

Baby's
Chiropractors have been treating children of all ages for more than a century. Chiropractic is effective and save for children. The treatment consists of light pressure techniques to correct blockades and cannot be compared to a treatment for adults.

Causes and complaints
During growth a child is faced with a great deal of physical stress. The first thing the spinal column encounters is the 'forced' position in the womb. Many women are familiar with the fact that foetal positions, like breech presentation or transverse presentation, can cause problems during delivery. Less well-known is that such positions can also affect the spinal column of the foetus. Even during a normal delivery a lot of pressure is being applied to the body of the baby. A Caesarean seems less traumatic but this is not the case. Symptoms of a new-born baby can be caused by irritation of the nervous system due to blockades in the back.

These symptoms may include
- Restless, nervous, a lot of crying
- Sleep problems/rhythm problems
- Preferred position of head or pelvis
- Extreme crying during dressing- and undressing
- Unstable head control for his/her age (the head follows slowly when the arms are raised)
- Retarded development (especially with regard to locomotion)
- Constipation.

Of course these symptoms may also have a different cause. The chiropractor assesses whether treatment is required.

Symptoms
At least fifteen percent of new-born babies cry excessively and are inconsolable. The description of '*cry babies*' says that babies less than three months old cry at least three hours a day, more than three days a week, and more than three weeks consecutively, usually in the late afternoon or in the evening. All this crying may cause stress and disturb the relationship between mother and child. Crying is often the expression of pain, for example due to tummy troubles, allergies or blockades of the spinal column. It is often said that excessive crying will cease at around the age of three months. Blockades that affect development may still be present. That's why it is advisable to let children older than three months be examined by a chiropractor, especially when they cried a lot as a young baby.

A much mentioned problem in children is the syndrome of '*Headvertebrae Influence on Disturbances in Symmetry*. This syndrome includes a wide range of complaints that may occur in babies and children, including crying, preferred position, etc. Sometimes only vague symptoms are present. These complaints are caused by blockade in the region of the upper neck vertebrae and the undesirable adaptation of the body to this.

It is always necessary that the chiropractor examines the whole body since neck problems can also result from mobility limitations in the pelvis.

When children are growing up, starting crawling and walking, falls and little accidents are unavoidable. Older children are in contact sports and other hobby's. At school children sit in poorly adapted chairs and often have to carry heavy bags. Such loads may result in tightening the muscles in the neck or back and in blockades in the spinal column.

Children cannot be regarded as small adults. The symptoms children have, do not always refer to the affected region. Examples are headache and bellyache or a change in behaviour.

But the following symptoms too may be present
- Problems in development
- Abnormal crawling or no crawling at all
- Frequent falls, dragging one's leg or foot or walking with foot turned inwards or outwards
- Clumsiness (motor problems)
- Pain in the legs
- Scoliosis (curvature of the spine)

Of course not all problems result from blockades in the spinal column. The chiropractor will always decide whether treatment is indicated or not.

Children

In children, like in adults, symptoms related to the locomotor apparatus may arise. This may already occur during delivery, but especially in the early years when they grow up. Falls, small accidents, sitting in school for hours, and sport can cause such symptoms. Usually children recover quickly, but if the symptoms persist, these should be examined.

Symptoms
Children cannot always show where the pain is located and so it is important to know that this is often reported as head-or tummy complaints. Also, the behaviour can reveal that the child is feeling unwell, such as being overly tired or hyperactive. Reduced resistance can be accompanied by physical symptoms, especially when children have underlying conditions like asthma, frequent throat-, nose- and ear complaints as well as scoliosis (curvature of the spine).

These conditions cannot be cured by the chiropractor but their effects can be limited, enabling the child to develop as much as possible 'as a child'. An example: children with asthma mainly employ chest breathing. This can result in heightened muscle tension in the shoulder area, accompanied by joint blockades in the upper back, from ribs to neck.

Treatment
The treatment of children differs from that of adults. Physical examination is carried out after an extensive interview with the child and the parents, after which the treatment can be started. Chiropractic corrections are attuned to children and are virtually painless.

In general children recover more quickly than adults and so the treatment frequencies are often lower, but this depends on the symptoms and the patient. The chiropractor proposes a personal treatment schedule.

Pregnancy

Chiropractic can be a real boon for a pregnant woman. A 'big tummy' is no obstacle to treatment, even towards the end of pregnancy. Besides it is safe for the developing child growing in the womb.

Causes of symptoms
It is not unusual that women get symptoms in the back or pelvic area. This is due to changes in hormone levels, increase in body weight and changes in posture. If the symptoms arise early during pregnancy or increase over time this can due to a problem in the functioning of the pelvis or spinal column. It is then advisable to see a chiropractor in order to let the pregnancy pass off smoothly.

Symptoms
Back symptoms during pregnancy are often due to the changed position of the pelvis. Since the child grows bigger and heavier, the downward force at the front of the spinal column steadily increases, resulting in the pelvis tilting forward and the lower back getting more

hollow. This causes irritation of the joints between the vertebrae, tense muscles and, so, pain.

This pain may be localized or radiate to the legs, the so-called pregnancy sciatica.

Chiropractic can improve the functioning of the lower back and pelvis and at the same time ensure maximal space in the abdominal cavity. Moreover, chiropractic improves the function of the pelvis and so the preparation for delivery.

Pelvis instability
Instability of the pelvis often occurs during pregnancy. Pelvis instability causes pain around the pelvis joints and the pubis due to the production of a hormone which relaxes the joint ligaments in the trimester of pregnancy. Sometimes this can cause hypermobility of the joints, through which the ligaments around the pelvis are no longer able to properly carry the body weight. In most cases the muscles can counterbalance this but if the muscle do not receive the right guidance from the nervous system pelvis instability can arise. Women experience pain around the tail bone, pubis or radiating pain to the legs when sitting, standing, walking and ultimately also when lying down.

Treatment
The chiropractic treatment for pelvis instability differs from the treatment of a blocked pelvis. In the case of pelvis instability the pelvis moves too much and the objective is to stabilize it by means of corrections and exercises and the optimal functioning of the nervous system and muscles. Because of its healing action on

the nervous system chiropractic can also be helpful in other areas, for example extreme nausea.

Sport injuries

Whether one goes in for sport for pleasure or professionally, every sportsman/sportswoman runs the risk of getting injured. Every year many get injured in sport; this is painful and annoying for the sportsman/sportswoman and expensive for society because of the considerable sickness absence due to injuries.

Prevention
Many sportsmen /sportswomen, holiday-makers and professionals, therefore opt for visiting a chiropractor regularly for a check-up. Experience shows that this preventive approach leads to a huge decrease in the number of injuries. Also soccer players turn out to be able to perform much longer.

Chiropractors
Chiropractors are ideally suited to treat or prevent problems involving muscles and joints. A well- functioning locomotor apparatus results in better performance and fewer injuries. Studies and experience show that the preventive approach of the chiropractor can drastically reduce the number of injuries. It also turns out that an active approach after an injury can strongly speed up revalidation.

Acute and chronic
Injuries can arise immediately or gradually. Immediately as a result of a sudden wrong movement and

gradually as a result of wrong movements which, perhaps, has crept in long ago. Of course it is desirable to treat these causes as soon as possible.

Symptoms
Diminished performance, slight pain or stiffness, or a slow recovery after minor injuries may indicate poor functioning muscles and joints. Even recurring knee- and ankle problems can be caused by an incorrect motion pattern in the lower back or hip.

Treatment of sportsmen/sportswomen
People engaged in sports demand a different approach, since the forces acting on the body in sports are so much greater than in daily life. A sportsman /sportswoman therefore must continue to rehabilitate longer after sustaining an injury; almost symptom-free is not good enough. A well-functioning body is characterized by the correct balance with respect to power, stamina, flexibility and coordination. Only then the sportsman/sportswoman has full control over his/her body and gets to know his/her potentialities and limitations.

Treatment
During the treatment the emphasis is on removing the blockades and restoring the mobility of muscles and joints. The chiropractor has numerous techniques at his disposal. He can also offer advice with regard to exercises and diet.

Source: Nederlandse Chiropratoren Assiociatie

18. Vertebrae, intervertebral disks and possible complaints

'The nervous system is designed to exert full control over organs and organ functions'

When vertebrae and/or intervertebral disks are shifted the nervous system can be affected. Spinal cord segments correspond to organs and organ functions; the complaints and symptoms that may arise when these segments are blocked are shown with the help of figure 3.

Spinal cord Segments	Corresponding organs/organ functions	Possible complaints
1C	Blood supply to the head, mucosae, scalp, cheek-bones, brain, ear organs, sympathetic nervous system	Headaches Nervousness Insomnia Colds High blood pressure Migraine Nervous breakdown Memory loss Dizziness Chronic fatigue

Spinal cord Segments	Corresponding organs/organ functions	Possible complaints
2C	Eyes, optical nerves, auditory nerves, nose and pharynx, ear bones, tongue, forehead	Nose and throat comcomplaints Dizzy spells Allergies Squint Deafness Eye problems Earache (sometimes) Blindness
3C	Cheeks, outside the ear, cheekbones, teeth, facial nerves	Neuralgia Neuritis Acne Eczema
4C	Nose, lips, mouth, Eustachian tube	Inflammation of mucosa Tonsillitis Hay fever
5C	Vocal cords, neck glands,	Laryngitis Angina Hoarseness
6C	Neck muscles, shoulders, tonsils	Tonsillitis Croup Pertussis Stiff neck Pain in the upper arms

Spinal cord Segments	Corresponding organs/organ functions	Possible complaints
7C	Thyroid gland, bursae in shoulders and elbows	Bursitis Colds Thyroid problems
1T	Gullet and windpipe, wrists, hands and fingers	Pain in under arms under arms, Asthma Cough Respiratory problems Shortness of breath
2T	Coronary artery, heart, heart valves	Heart complaints and other chest problems
3T	Chest, pleura, lungs, bronchi	Pneumonia Bronchitis Pleuritis Congestion Flu
4T	Gallbladder	Gallbladder complaints Shingles Jaundice
5T	Liver, blood, Plexus solaris	Low blood pressure Arthritis Poor circulation Liver complaints Fevers Anaemia

Figure 3

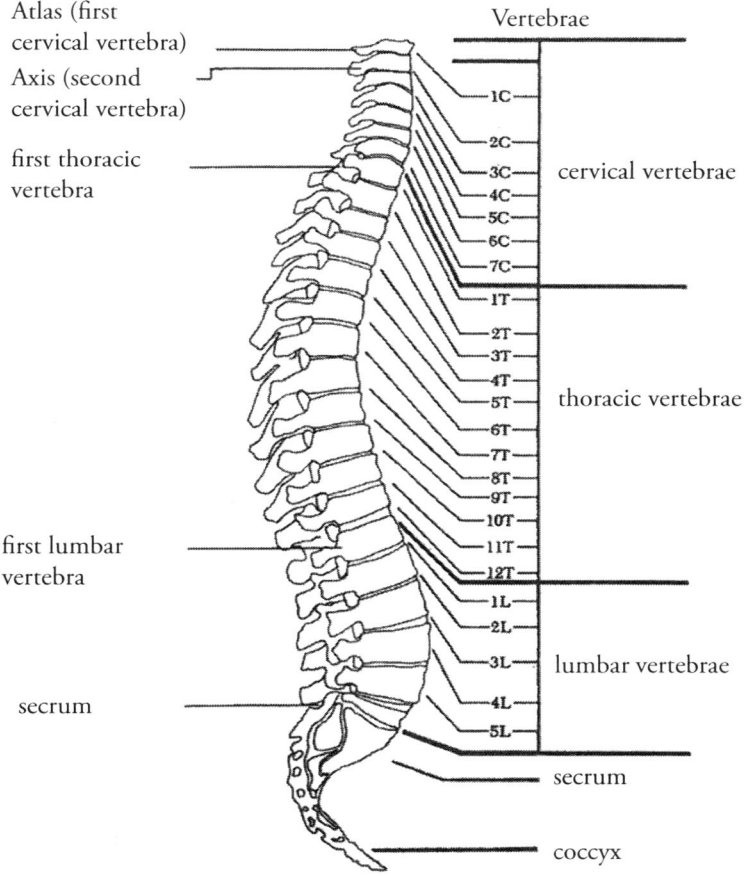

Spinal cord Segments	Corresponding organs/organ functions	Possible complaints
6T	Stomach	Digestion problems Stomach complaints Heartburn Indigestion
7T	Pancreas duodenum	Inflammation of gastric wall Ulcer formation
8T	Spleen	Lowered resistance
9T	Adrenals, located on top of kidneys	Allergies
10T	Kidneys	Kidney complaints Kidney inflammation Pyelitis Chronic fatigue Hardening of arteries
11T	Kidneys, ureters	Boils Pimples Eczema Skin complaints
12T	Small intestine, lymph circulation	Rheumatism Some forms of sterility

Spinal cord Segments	Corresponding organs/organ functions	Possible complaints
1L	Large intestine, groin area	Constipation Inflammation of large intestine Diarrhoea Bloody diarrhoea
2L	Appendix, belly upper legs	Respiratory problems Heartburn Varicose veins Cramps
3L	Urinary passages, sexual organs, knees	Bladder complaints Menstrual disorders Impotence Miscarriage Bed-wetting Knee pains Signs of old age
4L	Prostate, sciatic nerve, muscles in lower back	Hip gout Backache Pain at urinating
5L	Lower legs, feet, ankles	Poor circulation in the legs Weak legs Leg cramps Swollen ankles Cold feet Fallen arches

Spinal cord Segments	Corresponding organs/organ functions	Possible complaints
Sacrum	Hip bones, buttock	Curvature of the spine Ilium complaints Sacrum complaints
Tailbone	Rectum, anus	Pain while sitting Piles Itching

19. What chiropractic is not

*'In particular 'assumed similarities' with other
forms of treatments are a source of confusion.
Chiropractic is often confused with manual'*

Despite the increasing familiarity with chiropractic there is still confusion about this valuable therapy. It is thus important to throw some light on the greatest misunderstanding around chiropractic, viz. *'supposed similarities with other forms of treatment'*. For instance, chiropractic is often confused with manual therapy or with osteopathy.

Patients and persons involved think it concerns the same therapy. This is incorrect. Chiropractic and the therapies mentioned differ in all possible ways, both with regard to the underlying theory and principles as well as to the mode of treatment. So, it is useful to explain the essence of the other therapies.

Osteopathy
In chapter 15, *The training of the chiropractor,* we have mentioned that one of the subjects is *osteology,* the science of bones. In view of his vision on health and disease knowledge of bones is essential for the chiropractor. Osteopathy is a method based on the science of bones. Osteopathy is a so-called manipulative therapy. The term *osteopathy* is derived from the words *'osteon'* which means bone and *'patos'*

which is the Greek word for disease. The term osteopathy by itself is a source of confusion for it suggests that it refers to diseases of the bones. And that is incorrect. It does refer to a therapy that posits that bones / skeleton have a lot to do with illness and health. Naturally the spinal column plays a central role in this system.

The Greek and the Romans were very much interested in the physical structure and discovered that a poorly functioning locomotor system was probably the cause of many disorders. The American Dr. Andrew Still elaborated on this fundamental notion .Still (1828 – 1917) had a versatile mind.

He had studied architecture and medicine and was very religious. But he suffered much misfortune in his life, including the death of his three children who died of meningitis. Because his children could not be saved he took an aversion to conventional medical science.

On the basis of his studies, his faith and his disillusion with science Still developed a method which he called *machine theory*. In his opinion many disorders that had no apparent connection with bones yet result from a defect of the locomotor system.

Andrew Still was convinced that the human body was created by God and should never be seen as an accidental *collection of organs*. He believed there should be a connection, that all organs depended on each other and that the proper functioning of the locomotor system definitely exerted its influence on that. In a certain sense Still thus looked upon the body as a *machine*. When a machine isn't working properly it means that a part malfunctions, he argued. 'The whole machine then stops functioning properly.'

> *'The blood produces the necessary substances to give the body immunity and also to enable the body to defend itself against diseases'*

He even posited that man never could have been created to walk upright. By walking erect our vertebrae became weight-bearing, a function they were not designed for. According to Still walking upright caused disorders such as constipation, hernia, varices, etc. Further, Still believed that a well-functioning blood circulation is essential for the optimal condition of the body. The blood produces essential substances to give the body immunity and fight diseases.

Straight chiropractic

Straight chiropractors are those mainly focused on locating and correcting the 'subluxation' They don't in general make a real clinical diagnosis and in their interpretation of the field they stick to the original theories of D.D. Palmer. They feel very strongly about the underlying philosophy and their treatment is largely confined to manipulation techniques. This group makes little use of therapeutic exercises and myofascial treatment techniques*. Moreover this group claims that the effectiveness of the treatment also applies to general symptoms. According to the straight chiropractors almost every disease is caused by disturbances in the spinal column, a point of view that may have been plausible in 1895, but is no longer valid today.

* Myofascial therapy is directed towards the treatment of symptoms of posture and the locomotor system

---

On the basis of this view Still developed a method based on *osteopathic injuries*. Such an injury can be a joint where something is wrong, for example a shifted joint. Or a painful joint resulting from thickening of connective tissue. Further, swellings or other painful spots may be present. Such an osteopathic injury has seemingly nothing to do with the pattern of complaints. Yet this can result in a disturbance of the blood circulation whereby the organs are no longer optimally supplied with the required substances to enable the body to defend itself (the immune system). The injury can also result in an imbalance of the locomotor system while many other functions are affected, such as respiration, blood pressure and heart beat. This can lead to a chain reaction leading to a vicious circle unless the basic cause is tackled, the so-called osteopathic injury.

The osteopath tries to restore the original structure
Muscles, bones and joints are palpated by the osteopath. Or X-ray pictures are ordered. Connective tissue receives special attention. Thickenings, painful spots and swellings of the connective tissues are identified. The history and lifestyle are taken into account at establishing the cause of the injuries. Working conditions, living conditions, eating habits, etc. may have been contributing factors. When the mechanical disturbance (the injury) has been identified, and when the therapist knows the underlying cause, treatment can be started.

The joints are manipulated with the hands. The osteopath tries to restore the original structure in the joint or the painful spot. If he is successful the locomotor system too will be healed. In principle the osteopath claims to be able to treat the same complaints as other manual therapists. But the difference in view should be clear by now: the osteopath does not mention the harmful effect on the nervous system. And in chiropractic this is the all-embracing foundation for healing and health.

We will not pass judgment on osteopathy and definitely will not declare that chiropractic is superior to osteopathy. It concerns a very different view, an outlook which has nothing to do with chiropractic. But we should not fail to mention that it has been scientifically established that the nervous system controls the whole body. And this is not a basic assumption of osteopathy.

Manual medicine

Chiropractic is often wrongly identified with manual medicine. But this is unjustified. This - like in the case of osteopathy- results from the fact that manual medicine too attempts to restore defective joint functions. Obviously, with that too the spinal column is of central importance. But even when the spinal column occupies a place within a therapy this does not necessarily constitute a form of chiropractic. Contrary to chiropractic, which was developed in the 19th century, in most countries manual medicine has been developed relatively recently.

Manual medicine is not based on a specific view on sickness and health like in osteopathy and chiropractic. One maintains an open mind with respect to other existing treatments.

'But one is not very much concerned with the
possible cause, but one only establishes the
presence of a joint blockade and treats it'

When joint blockade is present then a decreased mobility of the joint will be present and its freedom of movement will be impaired. This may give rise to various complaints that are initially not recognized as being related to joint blockade. Various symptoms can be the cause of joint blockade. But one is not too much concerned with the possible cause, but simply determines that joint blockade is present and treats it.

The physical examination is focussed on the joints, the respiratory tract and the digestive tract. Muscles are examined and X-ray pictures are taken Also lab tests on blood and urine may be ordered.

Naturally the aim of the therapy is to remove the joint blockade. During this treatment joint surfaces are briefly separated from each other and other manipulations are performed to remove the blockades. Everything is done with the hands and the treatment is usually painless.

To summarize: manual medicine is a combination of other manual methods. The view concerning the cause is lacking to a certain extent. Of course one does have a view about disease and health and possible underlying causes, but these views are not clearly defined, while the manual therapist himself is of the opinion that these are unproven. The starting point is the 'actual' complaint and this is treated without further ado. The treatment can be executed by regular doctors and regular drugs may be prescribed. Manual therapists claim that many complaints respond well to the treatment, including neck/back-ache and eczema.

Here too we pass no judgment about the merits of this therapy but warn the reader that synthetic drugs may be prescribed, which is not the case in chiropractic. On the basis of this and the lack of a clear vision in manual medicine we still give preference to chiropractic.

> **Mixed chiropractic**
> The 'mixed' chiropractors represent the modern version. They mix other techniques in their therapy, seek to establish a clinical diagnosis whenever possible, and do not limit themselves exclusively to correcting subluxations. Indeed, the terms 'subluxation' and 'innate intelligence' (life force) from Palmer's original theories are considered unscientific and incomplete by this group. Mixed chiropractors are open to professional dialogue with conservative doctors and have the ambition to establish a recognized position within the regular health care. Mixed chiropractors are more nuanced with respect to their claims about effectiveness and limit their field of activity to complaints of the locomotor system, like back complaints, neck –and headaches, sport injuries, etc. No claims are made about effectiveness with regard to organic conditions or other pathological processes.

Manual therapy: 'system-Sickesz'

This therapy developed by the Dutch physician, Mrs. Maria Sickesz (1923 – 2015) is sometimes confused with chiropractic and/or manual medicine. This is incorrect. Definitely the therapy has nothing in common with chiropractic, while Sickesz view underlying her system also has nothing to do with manual medicine.

Sickesz points out that after all the spinal column rests on the pelvis. As a result of various causes the pelvis may grow crooked or it may be crooked as a result of a sudden event, for example a fall, lifting a heavy load the wrong way, an accident, etc.

When the pelvis is crooked through whatever cause then a difference in leg length can arise. Then the equilibrium gets out of balance resulting in an unnatural posture through which muscles get overloaded and nerves get wedged. This in its turn affects the spinal column and the ribs. This may cause complaints like backache, neck-ache, headache, pain in the shoulders etc. while at a later stage other complaints may occur. In this therapy too symptoms are mentioned that don't lead one to suspect that a crooked pelvis is connected with them.

The therapy implies that the correction is applied *to the pelvis*. Each rib is loosened which is done with the forefinger. The Sickesz-therapist is not so much looking for a stuck rib but treats all ribs and vertebrae and this is deemed necessary in order to correct the crooked pelvis. When one doesn't treat all ribs and vertebrae the complaints might return in the course of time. The treatment is painless as follows from the above. The therapy is often associated with the use of regular medicines. That is, when the complaint cannot be treated without the use of drugs. The Sickesz method also treats mental problems like depression, headache caused by mental problems, anxieties, etc.

Sickesz has found on the basis of her studies that forty percent of all (still) healthy individuals go through life with a crooked pelvis. According to her theory complaints lay lurking in this group. In patients - individuals with physical complaints- this percentage is much higher, something that quickly can be shown by measuring leg length. When there is a difference, a few millimetres or more, than crookedness has been established.

From the above it follows that the Sickesz-therapy has nothing in common with chiropractic. The fact that in both treatments the spinal column is the focus of attention makes no difference.

Manual therapy: 'system Van der Bijl'
The *system Van der Bijl* can be regarded as being derived from manual medicine. Van der Bijl developed a new therapy out of dissatisfaction with the existing therapies.

Van der Bijl (1909-1977) assumed the existence of '*deforming and reforming forces*'. Deforming forces are forces that disturb 'form' and can cause deformation, while reforming forces attempt to oppose it. Only when these two forces are perfectly balanced a state of perfect health can exist. There should be a constant interaction that exerts a great influence on the locomotor system. Further, Van der Bijl does not assume a certain fixed position of the spinal column. He thinks that that position is very personal and can differ among individuals. The position of the spinal column can be due to inherent properties or to acquired properties. So, Van der Bijl does not posit a dead straight position of the spinal column as the only correct position.

> *'Van der Bijl does not assume a certain fixed position of the spinal column. He believes that position is very personal and can differ among people'*

The position of the spinal column has much to do with the body's centre of gravity. Each body attempts to adapt itself to that centre of gravity in its own manner such that the pattern of movement (walking, standing) is unaffected. An adaptation that of course takes place subconsciously and over time. Still it can result in physical complaints at a later age. Van der Bijl attempts to determine which pattern of movement fits the patient best. In order to assess this the movements of the patient are observed. The way he/she walks, stands, sits, is of importance to establish a diagnosis. In fact Van der Bijl applies the theory of movement (kinesiology). The theory distinguishes 27 characteristic patterns of movement. He calls these patterns parameters. With the aid of these parameters the centre of gravity of the body is determined whether this centre of gravity fits the patient. When this is not the case corrections are made. This is done by little jolts of the hand. These are so gentle that the method is sometimes refer to as the '*eggshell-method*'. The jolts are so gentle that even an eggshell would not break. Van der Bijl claims that with this method the same complaints can be treated as those treated by the manual healer.

Final remark
The foregoing shows that chiropractic should not be confused with any of the other above-mentioned therapies. This will make the choice perhaps a bit simpler for the patient.

20. Preventing symptoms yourself

*'The well-known saying 'prevention is
better than cure' certainly holds
for the chiropractic view'*

The causes of complaints are often mentioned in this book. Many possible causes are beyond the control of the individual and we may assume that everybody is careful and tries to avoid a fall or an accident. But situations can arise through which one falls or gets involved in a car accident. We know that a fall, a thrust, a blow, or an impact can result in back-, neck, shoulder-, head complaints, etc. But on the other hand there are ways to prevent problems. The well-known saying *prevention is better than a cure* certainly holds for the chiropractic view. In this chapter some practical advice will be presented. Some of these tips will be easy to follow, others may perhaps require some change in lifestyle. Think that it is all about your health, which is worth 'protecting' above anything.

Preventing backache
Most complaints can be prevented by a proper posture. An incorrect posture can cause more complaints than one would think. For the rest an incorrect posture may be of long standing. If you can't correct it yourself it is advisable to seek the help of a chiropractor.

The following suggestions may be helpful to 'help yourself':

1. Try to be 'aware' when walking, sitting or exercising. Walk upright, relaxed and try to spread the body weight such that both feet bear the same weight.
2. Lounging in an easy chair increases tension on neck and shoulders. Try to sit straight in a proper chair with a straight back. If this is difficult, then alternate between an easy chair and a proper chair during a long evening.
3. Try as much as possible not to increase the natural curve at the lower end of the spinal column while sitting or standing. Sit and stand relaxed and try to assume a posture corresponding to the natural shape of the spinal column. One senses intuitively which posture feels best.
4. Don't use too many pillows when sleeping. One pillow for good support of neck and shoulders is sufficient for a good night's rest.
5. A firm matrass is essential as well as a natural position of the spinal column. There is no need for an expensive, custom-made matrass. An ordinary firm matrass is fine.
6. Avoid being overweight. Obese people suffer more from back complaints than others (*sand bag bending the bamboo pole*).
7. When lifting heavy objects don't bend but buckle under first, then grab the object and straighten up.

'Avoid being overweight. Obese persons suffer more from backache than others'

8. Spread the weight when carrying heavy objects as much as possible between both sides of the body. When the object is so heavy that you have to walk face forward the weight is really too heavy.
9. When gardening do not always bend over. It is better to kneel while trying to keep the back as straight as possible.
10. Never go in for sport without a trainer, never start the actual exercise without a 'warming up'. Never try to abruptly do heavy exercises or to achieve spectacular results.
11. A regular check-up by a chiropractor is advisable and can prevent a lot of trouble. If circumstances give cause a regular check-up - say, twice a year - should be considered.
12. Assume a proper posture while driving. Adjust the seat such that the head doesn't need to be stretched for a good view of the road. Obviously the seat should support the back properly. This prevents tension on the shoulders. Good head rests are also important.

Neck-, shoulder- and arm pain
Of course the above not only applies to backache prevention. These suggestions are also meant to avoid neck-, shoulder- and arm pain. With regard to neck and shoulders a few more hints:

1. Try to keep neck and back in a straight line. Avoid pushing the head forward or jutting out the chin while walking.

2. Avoid working over your head. Having to reach up with your arms over prolonged periods causes muscle pain.
3. Avoid working or sleeping in the draught. A good ventilation and fresh airflow is excellent, but it shouldn't be draughty.
4. Avoid getting overtired and try to rest on time. This holds especially for very demanding working conditions.
5. Make sure you get the right exercise. Go in the open air in your spare time. And remember, a walk during lunch hour is better than sitting in a hot canteen…
6. Peering at a computer screen causes headache and neck problems. It is essential to take a rest after two hours behind the computer. Rest your eyes and shoulders for a while.

Headache complaints and migraine
The following hints may help when you're suffering from headache or migraine:

1. When it is established that the nature of the headache is associated with certain foods or drinks these should be avoided. Even small quantities may cause complaints.
2. When the headache is caused by emotional stress let off steam by doing something else. Adequate relaxation prevents headache.
3. Just as with neck-and shoulder pains may be due to 'computer overload' the same is true for headache. It is very important to take a short break every hour.

4. Headache patients in particular should not use to many pillows while sleeping. One pillow should be sufficient. Proper neck support is essential.
5. Make sure your bedroom is well-ventilated. Sleeping in a too warm room is discouraged.
6. Sleeping on your stomach too may cause headache.
7. Do not work, sit or sleep in a draught. Driving with open windows - also in summer -produces draught. This may cause headache.

Closing remarks

Health is a very personal matter. There is no ready-made 'recipe' for a healthy life. The foregoing hints should be regarded as guidelines. Possibly they may be overlooked when searching for the cause of complaints. Each individual must decide for himself what is healthy for him/her and in what manner the lifestyle could be adjusted. When symptoms are present the first thing you've to do is try to identify the cause yourself. You shouldn't leave everything to the therapist or the doctor. For the cause too is personal. What is bothering one person may benefit the next. The first and most important point is that one should be aware of the cause. Once this 'awareness' is present the solution is close at hand.

21. Diet and health

*'Without our being aware of it we consume
many pounds of chemicals a year. No wonder
symptoms will arise sooner or later'*

No book about health and the prevention of symptoms should be without a chapter about diet and health.

We can safely state that proper diet is important for maintaining good health and that poor diet may lead to complaints. But at the same time diet is one of the most neglected factors. We often eat too much, at irregular hours, and consume too much fatty foods. Due to hamburgers and French fries more and more people are overweight, including children. Many studies have shown a relationship between poor diet and cancer.

With our food chemicals enter our body, such as the above - mentioned colourings - and flavourings and artificial odours. Also, chemicals to speed up the growth of crops, chemicals to kill or shoo away insects as well as drugs prescribed by the doctor, like tranquilizers and sleeping pills, are also ingested.

Without us being aware of it we consume pounds of chemicals a year. No wonder symptoms will arise sooner or later! Anyone who tries to live a healthy life, avoids smoking and alcohol, but eats poorly, is still not living a healthy life. Perhaps healthy food is the key to perfect and lasting health. In chiropractic this idea is emphasized and it is assumed that physical complaints are the direct effect of unhealthy food.

What exactly is poor and what is healthy food?
We mentioned the foodstuffs containing chemical substances. It is best to avoid these foods. It is harder to assess non-pre-packaged foods. The so-called health-shops offer at least more security by offering unsprayed fruit and vegetables, etc. Most (fatty) food in snack bars and fast food restaurants is not healthy.

Confectionary and other sweet things usually contain colourings- and flavourings. Apart from being unhealthy it also makes us fat. Being obese can be very detrimental to your health.

We also consume drinks containing colourings and flavourings. Lemonade contains colourings as well as many alcoholic drinks. There are yellow, blue, green and red liqueurs. All these different colours are due to the addition of chemicals.

Meat or no meat, that's the question…
Are we allowed to eat meat or not? There is no simple answer. There are many 'health- diets' available. A large number of these 'prohibits' the consumption of meat and the compilers are convinced that eating meat is bad for your health. Some, on the other hand, don't 'prohibit' its consumption, but state that humans don't need meat. Others argue that it is obvious that man is not a carnivore but a herbivore. Incidentally, the butcher's meat is, in most cases, also treat-

ed with chemicals. The consumer expects meat to be 'red' but this is usually not the case. That's why meat is given a colour, again with chemicals. In addition the living animal also is treated with chemical substances to stimulate growth.

So, meat is not essential and is considered by many in the '*world of health and disease*' as superfluous. But healthy eating is a personal matter. He who believes man is not able to do without meat is advised to eat little meat. A good alternative is fish and/or poultry (chicken) while there are many healthier meat-substitutes available. And remember that fish too may have lived in polluted waters, a sea of chemical waste…

> *So, meat is not essential and is regarded by many authorities in the world of health and disease as superfluous*'

Thus far we have considered the question concerning bad food. The next question is: what should I eat, what is healthy food? We'll attempt to answer this question. 'Attempt', because there are no cut-and-dried answers. For after all, many originators of health diets consider their diet is the only correct one. In any case these different diets can be regarded as useful pointers. But the only right diet is the one you put together on the basis of these pointers. It is no use trying to persuade someone to eat food he/she doesn't like.

Our advice is: 'eat what you enjoy but stick to the pointers that influence health positively'. Below we will discuss some health diets.

Bircher Benner- diet
The Swiss doctor Max Bircher Benner (1867-1939) believed man requires sun-energy. Plants grow when they receive sufficient sun-energy. Animals eat plants that grow by sun-energy. Taking this into account Bircher Benner did not categorically condemn the consumption of meat but he did not recommend it either. Bircher Benner further pointed out that with baking and cooking a lot of sun-energy is lost. Therefore he advised people to eat as much raw food as possible. Raw food brings the maximal amount of sun-energy into the body. As a doctor Bircher Benner prescribed his diet for his patients, especially for those suffering from stomach- or intestinal disturbances.

He also achieved good results with his diet in patients with various other complaints such as chronic fatigue, feeling unwell, headache and listlessness. His diet in fact boils down to a more healthy life-style, resulting in the prevention of symptoms. Fish and meat are allowed sparingly, but only if one finds it hard to eliminate it from the diet.

The Bircher Benner diet means in daily practice that at least half of the food should be eaten raw: fruit, grains, fresh vegetables, seeds. Apples are allowed, but unpeeled! Peeling removes a lot of sun-energy. Further, Bircher Benner advises to eat Muesli at breakfast each morning as well as an appetizer at dinner. Less well-known is the fact that Bircher Benner is the originator of the familiar muesli recipes. Two muesli recipes:

Muesli
- 3 table spoons water
- 1 table spoon oatmeal
- 200 grams apple
- 1 tablespoon sweet condensed milk
- 1 tablespoon grinded nuts

Applemuesli
- 3 tablespoons water
- 3 tablespoons yoghurt
- 1 tablespoon oatmeal (soaked overnight)
- 1 tablespoon honey
- 200 grams apple
- 1 tablespoon grinded nuts

Avoid as much as possible such products as sugar, salt, coffee, thee, chocolate, cacao, bouillon, meat, fish, hot spices, alcohol, nicotine and drugs. The Bircher Benner diet is recommended for life, but only if it agrees with you! It does take some doing – perseverance - to get used to it. But it is better to 'cheat' occasionally than to disregard this diet altogether.

The Bircher Benner diet is effective in the following conditions: stomach-ache and abdominal pains, constipation, indigestion, bloated stomach, fatigue, headache, exhaustion, loss of energy.

Mayr-cure
The Austrian physician Dr. Franz Mayr (1875-1965) is the originator of the Mayr-cure named after him. For the rest his view involves more than diet alone. His suggestions may be regarded as a kind of philosophy of life.

Mayr posits that our body fluids like blood, lymph and bile wash the body cells. When these body fluids are polluted disorders end illnesses arise. Just like the Bircher Benner diet de Mayr-cure is meant to prevent symptoms and if disease is present to bring about a cure.

As stated the Mayr-cure involves more than diet alone. According to Mayr his diet can only restore health when the *pre-cure* has been completed. The pre-cure is meant to 'clean ' possibly polluted body fluids. The diet will further 'clean up' these body fluids. Because of the many forms of pollution this thesis seems justifiable.

The pre-cure takes a few weeks:

- Sleep warm at night. The higher temperature will insure the disposal of pollutants by transpiration.
- Take a hot shower followed by a cold one in the morning.
- Right after getting up drink 250 cc tepid water with a spoonful magnesium sulfate. This stimulates the digestive tract.
- Brush the skin with a medium brush in the morning and in the evening. A couple of minutes is sufficient to achieve a better blood flow to the skin.
- No coffee, fatty foods, spices and drugs are allowed during the course.

> *'Thus Mayr deems it very important to reduce the number of meals per day from three to two'*

After following the pre-cure for two weeks the Mayr-diet can be started. It must however be pointed out that the diet requires a certain amount of perseverance. Thus Mayr deems it very important to reduce the number of meals per day from three to two. The main meal should be taken five to six hours after breakfast. Thus the digestive organs get enough rest between meals, especially during sleep and between the main meal and breakfast. Food taken just before sleep has too little time to be digested. So, don't eat anything before going to bed. Further Mayr recommends to chew consciously, preferably fifty times. Well pre-chewed food is well mixed with saliva and so the digestive tract has less difficulty digesting the food.

The diet
Mayr does not advise against the use of meat, but recommends grilled meats: chicken, veal- and beef. Also permitted are: cheese, boiled eggs, margarine, or plant oils instead of animal fats. Preferable to coffee is: mineralwater, lime-blossom thee, rose hip thee, camomile thee, lemon juice, orange juice and balm.

Mayer advises against: fried (baked) food, bread, pork, raw food (!), cauliflower and sweets.

During illness it is prudent to fast for a couple of days. For the rest, Mayr recommends an occasional fast for 24 hours also in health. Then the digestive tract is given rest. Apart from promoting health and preventing many symptoms the Mayr diet is recommended for abdominal disturbances, constipation, allergies, headaches, fatigue, rheumatism.

Macrobiotics
Erroneously the macrobiotic diet is often thought to be boring. There are a lot of misunderstandings about this diet. But the macrobiotic diet is part of an all-encompassing philosophy of life. Naturally a healthy diet should be part of it. Sometimes macrobiotics is referred to as a *non-religious religion.* Another misconception is that macrobiotics prohibits the use of meat. That too is not true. Macrobiotics does hold that man is not a carnivore by nature. Meat is allowed, but only sparingly. A lot can be said about macrobiotics and much has been written about this philosophy of life. Here we'll mention a few striking facts.

At least half of the main meal should consist of grains. Also, vegetables and seaweed should be eaten daily. This doesn't have to be boring. Consider that there are many kinds of grains, vegetables and seaweed. Examples are: buck weed, barley, rice, wheat, bulgur, rye, spelt, oat, oat flakes, maize, pasta (spaghetti and vermicelli).

Beans, too, are part of macrobiotics: adzuki beans (red soy beans), black and yellow soy beans. As a substitute for the common table salt Mediterranean sea salt is used, or tamari (soya sauce), miso (soya pasta) or umeboshi-prunes (salty prunes). For drinks is recommended grain tea), herbal tea and apple juice. In cookbooks you'll find hundreds of recipes. Apart from the recipes for breakfast, lunch and dinner you'll also find recipes for sweets and tasty but healthy snacks.

Eating and drinking differently
Above we have sketched out the main features of healthier food. There are no concrete directions and perhaps you will decide to mix different types of diet to suit your own preferences.

A brief discussion of sugar, salt, coffee, smoking, alcohol and bad eating habits is presented below.

Sugar
Few people realize that sugar is a poison for the human body. Sugar - the way we use it - is in fact superfluous. We consume too much sugar, added to our food, candy and other things. The body struggles daily against this overload of large quantities of refined sugar. The body also protests by stomach complaints, constipation, chronic colds, irritation pimples, etc. Sugar is directly taken up in the bloodstream resulting in a sharp increase in glucose. The pancreas instantly produces more insulin to lower the glucose level. It may even happen that too much insulin is produced, resulting in a sharp drop in blood glucose below its fasting level. The result is hypoglycaemia with its symptoms like faintness, profuse sweating, etc.

The body attempts to correct this by drawing on the natural stores of sugar in the body (stored in the liver as glycogen). This may lead to the exhaustion of the supply of sugar and vitamins. This may result in tiredness and a weakened immune system. Remember that the right food contains enough sugar - partly 'packaged' as carbohydrates - for the optimal functioning of the body. Adding refined sugar is unnecessary and very bad. If you do need some extra sugar add a small quantity of honey.

Salt
Salt is essential. That's a well-established fact. Salt regulates the metabolism. But this does not mean that our table salt is required for this. Household salt contains sodium chloride that has been chemically purified. Much better to use Mediterranean sea salt, available in health shops.

Coffee
We're so used to drinking several cups of coffee a day that we don't realize coffee is a drug, even an addictive drug, deleterious to your health. This may cause stomach complaints and worse still: damage to the nervous system resulting in (jittery) nerves. The desire for coffee is purely the result of addiction. Try to limit coffee drinking to one cup a day. Perhaps you can even stop drinking coffee and drink herb thee or spring water instead.

And other drugs?
Smoking cigarettes, cigars or pipe has been mentioned in passing above. Everyone knows smoking is bad. So, we'll skip this topic since everyone understands what grave damage it may cause (lung-, mouth- tongue cancer and many other diseases). Naturally that also applies to the misuse of alcohol which can lead to social- and physical problems. Better not drink alcohol or at most a glass of wine or cyder, or beer without sugar. Think that some drugs are also addictive.

Final note
We live fast and hurried lives, which is reflected in our eating habits. So, we eat hurriedly and forget the

body needs time to properly digest the food. Realize that the food we eat is 'later' turned into our flesh, bones and blood. Food is of vital importance.

'Be aware' when you're eating, eat slowly and chew thoroughly. Don't eat anything for at least four hours before going to bed, so, no snacks either. During rest the body needs more time to digest the food, otherwise food residues will stay behind in the stomach and intestines, resulting in complaints.

Leading a healthy life starts with eating healthy food, acquiring the habit of healthy eating and drinking, avoiding bad foods, no smoking and not too much alcohol. If you continue to eat bad food, smoke and drink too much jogging in the open air or exercise in a gym doesn't make much sense.

22. Breathing

*'There is another important aspect,
often overlooked, proper breathing'*

Proper food, proper exercise, proper body posture: factors that contribute to good health. We are - on reflection - fully aware of this. Still we do not give these factors sufficient attention.

There is another important aspect, often overlooked: proper breathing.

Breathing the wrong way can have consequences for our body posture, from which symptoms may arise. But what is improper and what is and proper respiration ?

A proper method is abdominal respiration, sometimes called *belly breathing. Chest breathing*, the superficial breathing, is the improper way. Psychotherapists state that will rising problems (stress) respiration rises from the belly to the chest. This leads to superficial breathing and may result in a lack of oxygen.

Oxygen

The body cells are then insufficiently supplied with oxygen. The body protests and frantically struggles to obtain sufficient oxygen. Respiration thus becomes a laborious matter and this can affect body posture.

Conversely poor body posture can affect the way we breathe. If you're weighted down by worries and stress body posture deteriorates leading to more difficult breathing. Some therapists believe that poor breathing can be the cause of a heart attack. In any case incorrect breathing can result in a number of complaints. As a result of fatigue resulting from poor breathing and/or poor body posture muscles may tighten. And we know that tense muscles may result in subluxations, not to mention the most common complaint: hyperventilation.

> '*Some therapists believe that poor
> breathing can be the cause of a heart attack*'

Yet it is simple to improve your breathing pattern. Improving body posture will result in improved breathing. The following exercise will help to improve your breathing, which may help to improve your body posture.

Exercise
Sit on a chair with a straight back and be aware of your breathing. When you breathe properly you'll notice that your chest hardly moves. That's clearly seen in babies who naturally breathe the right way. Be aware of this and attempt to consciously coordinate inhalation and exhalation. Inhale for three seconds and exhale for six seconds.

If you manage in the sitting position try it in other positions. First standing, then lying down, sitting, etc. If you do these exercises a few times a day, at home, in the train or at work you will notice that belly breathing will become automatic after a while. This will also be maintained during heightened activity, such as during heavy work or sports.

Complaints
With better breathing various complaints may disappear. Overall you'll be feeling better, which you will already notice when getting up in the morning. Stamina will improve and if you suffer from hyperventilation this complaint will also quickly disappear. Better respiration and better body posture have a favourable influence on stress-related complaints. Tense muscles relax and tiredness, chest pain and shortness of breath disappear. In case you do not succeed in improving your breathing you can always consult a chiropractor.

23. With nature together

'We may state that chiropractic is part of natural medicine'

This book has made clear that chiropractic is close to nature and that that no drugs are used. Chiropractic posits that nature has (in some cases) dropped off to sleep, thus temporarily 'losing' the inborn wisdom of the body to keep itself free from ailments and complaints. The chiropractor points this out to nature. Stir up that sleepy defence system. After the correction of the mechanical disturbance the body resumes its tasks and nervous impulses freely flow through the body; muscles are free and function optimally. The nervous system also functions optimally. The complaints are gone. All this means that we may state that chiropractic is part of natural medicine.

Concern about one's own life-style

From this it follows that nature may well be assisted occasionally, because we no longer live in accordance to nature's laws. Stronger still, we all live unnaturally, contrary to nature. Man is not created only to work hard, to be constantly under pressure, to watch TV for hours, to eat hamburgers. Of course we are exaggerating but it seems appropriate in this context. It is ok that the reader should be a bit concerned about his life-style and wonder how it can be improved.

Was it nature's intention that man should smoke, drink alcohol, use drugs and chemicals? And that man only toils and eats poorly? Everyone would agree that man is not meant for this. We may even wonder whether we are meant to eat meat. This may sound a bit moralistic but this is not our intention. We do ask for reflection, for reconsideration, where each may ask himself/herself some important questions concerning his/her own life-style.

> *'Was it nature's intention that man should smoke, drink alcohol, use drugs and chemicals?'*

In this book we have offered questions, suggestions and ideas. He who follows these hints and directions will at least take a few steps further down the road to better health. Realize a healthy life according to your own ideas. He who reflects will definitely arrive at the right ideas. Reconsideration means that one stops to consider what one does or doesn't do.

Reconsidering also means looking at one's life from a distance ('*helicopter-thinking*') and wonder if changes should be made.

Don't forget, a healthier life begins at home, in the office, workplace or wherever. Life begins with doing something positive a bit more or giving up something negative.

But there are no ready-made prescriptions for a healthy life. But there are instructions on how to develop 'awareness'.

Think positive
Start trying to think positive. Reflect daily for a couple of minutes on your own health. After getting up, or in the car in a traffic-jam, etc. Consider at the end of the day what happened that day. Try to distinguish the healthy factors from the unhealthy ones. You may be surprised to recall all the unhealthy things that happened that day or the day before. How much exercise did you take, how many cigarettes did you smoke? And what have you eaten that day? And how many glasses of alcohol?

Try to make this a daily routine. Maybe you will experience a slight anxiety, making you realize that things can't just go on like this, that you should eat less, stop smoking, drink less alcohol, take more exercise. That you should expose yourself less to stresses at work, including pressure of work. And that you should leave more to others, not trying to do everything yourself.

A few minutes reflection a day can lead to a healthier life.

These few minutes may lead to other things as well. Maybe you may want to get closer to nature. We have turned our back against nature and believe we can do without her. The question should be asked: is my life ready for a drastic reorganisation? What will happen if I continue in this way? Am I too heavy, too lazy, too unhealthy?

> *'When you find it hard to answer the
> question 'what is good and what is bad'
> it helps to visualize things'*

When you find it hard to answer the question 'what is good what is bad' it helps to visualize things. Look in your mind at your own body and regard it as an enterprise where you're employed. The enterprise doesn't run properly if it receives too few orders, if the backlog of orders is empty. But the business doesn't run properly either when the pressure of work is too high. The enterprise will collapse under the load and the same thing happens to the body. When the pressure is too high the body will collapse. In this context 'collapse' means: *the presence of disorders and symptoms.*

Try also to see the body as a home where you live. It you neglect to paint the house you will notice that will cracks appear. When you don't treat your body properly you will notice that sooner or later the body will protest. Or, take a look at a plant. A plant demands proper care, may be in dire need for water. When the plant does not receive proper care and water it dies.

So, that's visualizing, contemplating in peace and thinking positively. From that situation measures can be taken. Measures to take care of the body, to get closer to nature and re-establish contact with nature.

Opening the door to nature
When you try to develop that awareness try also to recall how long ago it was that you really admired a flower. How long ago was it to be grateful for some warmth of the sun, for a deep green grass. How long ago was it that one felt moved by watching young animals at play. He who wonders is already close to the solution; he who ponders the question already got the

key in his hand and simply has to open the door to nature.

'I have no time for that' is the standard excuse that is not acceptable. Everybody has time to reconsider and occasionally get closer to nature. Remember always, when reflecting on this theme, that you yourself are part of nature. That too is positive thinking! Be open for change. At home, at work, at play. Try to discover what is really enjoyable and what is definitely unpleasant. Seek ways to change the *unpleasant*. Try also to protect yourself against the unpleasant influences affecting you from outside. That won't be easy for we are daily swamped by bad news; in the newspapers and on television as well as at home and at work.

> *'Health has everything to do with the mind,*
> *our way of thinking, our way of accepting,*
> *our way of 'rejecting'*

Try to put things into perspective, by which you may well be a bit selfish. You don't have to be self-effacing all the time. Of course we're not alone in this world. But don't forget yourself. Your own existence, your own life. Health doesn't only concern your body. Health has everything to do with the mind, our way of thinking, our way of accepting, our way of 'rejecting'. But don't put the limit too high. He who thinks positively will not be affected by all kind of influences.

Disease must also be seen as a warning
We have too much blind faith in 'modern medicine'. When you're ill you will get help and be cured. Maybe

that is true. We hope so in any case. But the illness must also be seen as a warning. However serious or however mild the symptoms may be. Life after the illness must be different from before.

In fact we have forgotten why we seek help from a healer. That is not only to be cured. It is also the remain *permanently* healthy after the complaint or the illness.

That doesn't happen just like that. We must stop living from one complaint to the next. From one healer to the next. And then continue in our old ways. That's asking for trouble, for new problems, sooner or later. We have to learn from an illness or complaint. To become convinced that something is wrong the way we live. So something should be done about it! So, develop a greater awareness, 'positive thinking', reconsidering. And try to live a better life after a complaint.

> *'Develop a greater awareness, 'positive thinking', reconsidering, try to live a better life after a complaint'*

Hopefully the disorder was just a warning. A cry from nature. Shake nature's hand and go on living, but now differently! Better! Healthier, making sure you won't be needing healers any more, nor regular doctors, nor chiropractors. If you won't listen you'll be needing another warning, a 'repeat illness'. But nature will not go on forever broadcasting warnings. The moment may arrive that we're struck with an incurable disease.

Think positive, develop that state of mind, and return to nature. When the disease is gone remember it will be the first day of the rest of your life. Be thankful that nature is giving you a second chance.

'Shake hands with nature and go on living, but now differently! Better! Healthier!'

24. Most frequently asked questions about chiropractic

1. Is chiropractic a new form of treatment?
Chiropractic as it is applied today is about a hundred years old. That implies that chiropractic is indeed a new form of treatment. But it should be realized that five thousand years ago healings were performed that strongly resemble current chiropractic.

2. Do you need a referral letter from the doctor to see a chiropractor?
No. Everyone with complaints can make an appointment with a chiropractor. Without referral letter. It may happen that an insurer demands such a letter.

3. How long does a treatment take?
It differs from one patient to the next and depends on the nature and seriousness of the complaint. Sometimes the complaint improves after a single treatment of a hour, but in most cases a series of six to ten treatments is required.

4. Is the treatment expensive?
The first visit can be a bit more expensive than the follow-ups. The first visit takes longer because of the exhaustive examination and possibly the chiropractor will request an X-ray. Te The treatment is certainly not expensive.

5. Can the treatment be dangerous?
No, a treatment is not risky. The chiropractor only uses his hands. Drugs and/or operations are not used. When it turns out that the chiropractor is unable to treat the specific complaint he refers the patient to another therapist, doctor or specialist. Of course the patient should check if the chiropractor has completed his training.

6. Does it work?
It sometimes happens that the patient notices an improvement or less pain immediately after the treatment. But it may also happen that one feels less well for a short period of time. This is a normal and positive reaction. It means that the complaint responds to the treatment. After a couple of treatments the patient will surely feel better.

7. What does the chiropractor do if he is unable to help?
In such a case the chiropractor refers the patient to another therapist, doctor or specialist. Thanks to his training the chiropractor is able to establish a correct diagnosis, also for complaints that he himself is unable to treat.

8. Can you only consult a chiropractor when you have complaints?
Definitely no. A chiropractor concentrates on the prevention of complaints. A regular visit to the chiropractor, say, twice a year for a check-up is highly recommended. This holds for everyone but in particular for children, older people, sportsmen /sportswom-

en and people in jobs involving heavy physical work. (Ex) patients too are advised to regularly visit the chiropractor for check-ups.

9. Is a chiropractor only meant for adults?
Chiropractic is for everybody, both for treating symptoms and for prevention. Children often horse about wildly and thus run the risk of injuring their vertebrae. It is therefore important that parents occasionally have their children checked by a chiropractor. This may prevent trouble in later years.

10. Can the chiropractor treat sports injuries?
The chiropractor also treats complaints resulting from sports. In the US top sportsmen and sportswomen often have their own 'personal chiropractor'. Sport and chiropractic go together.

11. Is the treatment painful?
Usually the patient will hardly feel anything. Sometimes the chiropractor exerts a bit extra pressure on the vertebrae or joints. This can be felt, but is definitely not painful.

12. Can the complaints return after the treatment?
It is best to return from time to time for a check-up. It sometimes happens that the advice of the chiropractor is not sufficiently complied with, which may result in the complaint returning.

13. Are drugs prescribed?
No, chemical drugs are not prescribed. Vitamins and minerals are sometimes suggested. The chiropractor

will offer advice about better food, since poor food can also lead to symptoms.

14. I have been referred to the physiotherapist for my backache. Is the chiropractor better?

The physiotherapist treats backache usually with exercises and correcting body posture. Sometimes massage is used. The physiotherapist is a competent therapist but the chiropractor operates from a very different point of view, a view that goes deeper and is especially focussed on the proper functioning of the nervous system.

15. Are doctors opposed to chiropractic?

No, doctors are not opposed to chiropractic but regular doctors usually stick to 'regular'. But the number of doctors that recognize the value of chiropractic and refers the patient to the chiropractor is growing.

16. Can the chiropractor cure cancer?

The chiropractor makes no such claim and will never tell the patient to be able to cure cancer. Yet, he may be able to alleviate the pain caused by cancer or other diseases.

17. How do I find a reliable chiropractor

A reliable chiropractor is a chiropractor who has completed a stiff study. He may then call himself *doctor of chiropractic.* If you have doubts about his training you can contact one of the organisations mentioned at the end of this book.

18. How do I know I have to see a chiropractor?
You can see a chiropractor for a great number of different complaints. Most complaints have been mentioned in various earlier chapters. See in particular chapter 17 (*Summary: 'which complaints'*).

19. What advice may I expect from the chiropractor?
Depending on the nature and the severity of the complaints the chiropractor will offer advice with regard to a better environment, posture, exercise, diet, life-style and/or a healthier way of sitting or lying down.

20. Does the chiropractor have anything in common with manual medicine and/or osteopathy?
Manual medicine and osteopathy are different methods with a different underlying view. De way of treatment is also totally different. The differences have been discussed in this book (see chapter 20: '*What chiropractic is not*').

21. Does chiropractic go together with other treatments like acupuncture and homeopathy?
It is possible that in some cases this is open to objection. Much depends on the nature of the complaint. It may also be unnecessary to call in another therapist. Please consult with your chiropractor.

22. Do health insurers refund the treatment?
Usually health insurers refund the treatment, possibly on the basis of supplementary insurance.

23. Where can you get help if you have complaints about a chiropractor?

In such cases you can turn to the Chiropractic Patients Federation Europe or the Anglo-European College of Chiropractic. The addresses are found at the end of this book.

24. Is there a patients' association?

The Chiropractic Patients Federation Europe. The address is presented at the end of this book.

25. Can you prevent backache yourself?

Definitely you can do a lot to prevent back complaints. Practical advice is given in chapter 21 ('*Preventing symptoms yourself*'). When you're being treated by a chiropractor you can be assured that he will offer you practical advice to prevent back trouble and other complaints in the future.

26. Is it better not to see a chiropractor when you are pregnant?

On the contrary. Especially the expectant mother runs a higher risk of back complaints. During a couple of months a 'heavy load' must be carried. The chiropractor can help the expectant mother with regard to back complaints and other complaints and make sure the symptoms do not recur. The chiropractor can offer the mother advice during pregnancy and after delivery. Advice for both mother and child.

Glossary

The most commonly used terms in chiropractic

Adjustment
A treatment which the chiropractor executes to correct blockades in the vertebral segments, by which disturbances in the nervous system can be removed.

Alternative medicine
A therapeutic mode starting from a different view of disease and health than regular medicine. Also (in most cases) a different mode of treatment is employed. Alternative medicine is not recognized by the authorities.

Autonomic nervous system
That part of the nervous system responsible for the so-called 'automatic body processes', like digestion, sex organs, blood vessels and excretory organs.

Chiropractic
A holistic form of treatment (see *Holism*) aimed at promoting general health, or to restore and support it by removing communication disturbances in the function of the nervous system by application of dosed mechanical impulses.

Chiropractor
A therapist who practices chiropractic.

Foramina intervertebralia
The openings between the vertebrae through which the nerves run.

Functional chiropractic
Also referred to as neuro-physiological chiropractic or modern chiropractic. Functional chiropractic attempts to locate where the nervous system does not function properly and is less focused on the theory of crooked vertebrae and such (subluxations). See also 'structural chiropractic'.

Holism (holistic medicine)
The view that holds that the phenomenon of life is determined by the value of its totality and not by its parts.

Innate intelligence
This is meant to express the wisdom of the body to protect itself against disease and to heal itself.

Intervertebral disks
Elastic disks of cartilage between two vertebrae. These act as shock absorbers, so the shocks don't have to be absorbed by the vertebrae themselves.

Manual therapy
A therapy exclusively executed with the hands, thus, a treatment does not involve the use of drugs, radiation or operation.

Migraine
In the case of migraine a sudden sharp headache may be accompanied by nausea and vomiting. Also hyper-

sensitivity to light and sound is present. Migraine occurs when the blood vessels in the brain first constrict, then dilate. The cause is unknown.

Motion palpation
Within this context it refers to palpating the spinal column. By this the chiropractor locates the subluxation. There are two different forms of palpation. The 'motion palpation' is performed with the patient in different positions while standing, sitting or lying down. See also 'Static palpation'.

Motor nerves
Nerves that control locomotion of the organism.

Nerve signals
Stimuli transmitted by the nerves to the organs and tissues. Without these signals the organs and tissues don't function properly.

Nervous system
Where the 'nervous system' is mentioned in this book it refers to the central nervous system, the brain and the spinal cord.

Parasympathetic nervous system
Part of the autonomic nervous system that influences organs in such a way that the body can be in a condition of rest and recovery.

Peripheral nervous system
Peripheral means on the outside. So, the peripheral nervous system is the nervous system at the

periphery of the body that connects the central nervous system with the rest of the body. (see also Nervous system).

Psychosomatics
The study and treatment of physical disorders caused by mental problems.

Regular Medicine
This the 'normal' medicine taught at the university (as practiced by doctors, specialists, dentists).

Sensory nerves
The nervous system is functionally connected with the organism and the environment.

Spinal column
The spinal column or backbone consists of a number of bones that protect the spinal cord and enables us to walk upright. The greatest part of the body is 'supported' by the spinal column. Further, the spinal column is of critical importance for the proper functioning of the nervous system.

Spinal cord
The cord of 32 pairs of nerves running through the hollow space of the vertebrae from the cerebellum to the lumbar vertebrae. The spinal column encloses the spinal canal through which the spinal cord runs. A fluid, the cerebrospinal fluid) runs through the spinal cord, which plays a major role in the signalling of nerve signals.

Static palpation
Here palpation mean: palpating (feeling) the spinal column. The 'static palpation' is performed when the patient is lying down. See also 'Motion palpation'.

Stress
Mental problems that exerts a negative influence on the proper functioning of the body and may lead to physical complaints.

Structural chiropractic
Also referred to as biomechanical chiropractic or the classical method. Structural chiropractic looks for deviations in the position of the vertebrae and other body parts. Such a deviation is called a subluxation (see below).

Subluxation
This term refers to a crooked position of a vertebra which causes a disturbance in the nervous system.

Sympathetic nervous system
Part of the autonomic nervous system. The automatic nervous system operates on our subconscious level. That means that we are unable to influence it with our 'conscious will'. It operates automatically as its name indicates. The automatic nervous system consists of the sympathetic nervous system and the parasympathetic nervous system, which, a bit like our flexor and extensor muscles of the thigh, work together 'antagonistically'.

Total diagnosis
A complete and thus extensive diagnosis.

Traditional medicine
Knowledge and practices used in treatment and prevention developed over generations before the era of modern medicine.

Below are listen the books on health and medicine written by Robert Jan Blom

- Chiropractie als alternatief (NL)
- 25 Alternatieve geneeswijzen (NL)
- Gezondheid van dag tot dag (NL)
- Alternatieve geneeswijzen (NL)
- 35 Alternatieve geneeswijzen (NL)
- Acupunctuur (NL)
- Homeopathie (NL)
- Macrobiotiek (NL)
- Alternative Heilmethoden (German)
- Chiropractie, de derde geneeskunde (NL)
- Wegwijzer alternatieve geneeskunde (NL)
- Chiropraktik (German)
- Sanft Heilen (German)
- Natuurlijk beter worden (NL)
- Chiropractie (NL)
- Je Lichaam afstaan aan de Wetenschap (NL)
- Fobieën, Angsten en Dwangneuroses (NL)
- What Chiropractic can do for you (English)

Addresses

Anglo-European College of Chiropractic (AECC)
Bournemouth **www.aecc.ac.uk**

Belgium **www.chiropraxie.org**
Germany **www.chiropraktik.de**
France **www.chiropratique.org**
The Netherlands **www.nca.nl**
United Kingdom **www.chiropractic-uk.co.uk**
UK General Chiropractic Council **www.gcc-uk.org**

Chiropractic Patients Federation Europe
www.prochiropractic.org

Lectures and journalistic contributions:

Robert Jan Blom (Author)
Aletta Jacobsstraat 69
2401 KL Alphen aan den Rijn
The Netherlands

Email: rj.blom01@hetnet.nl
Tel. 00 31 654 917076
http://nl.wikipedia.org/wiki/Robert_Blom